Jordan's Voice

Jordan's Voice

THE LIFE OF AN UNDERDOG
How Bullying Affected the Lives of a Father and Son

Bradley L. Lewis

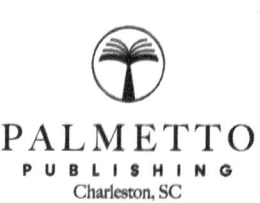

PALMETTO
PUBLISHING
Charleston, SC
www.PalmettoPublishing.com

Copyright © 2024 by Bradley L. Lewis

All rights reserved

No portion of this book may be reproduced, stored in a retrieval system, or transmitted in any form by any means—electronic, mechanical, photocopy, recording, or other—except for brief quotations in printed reviews, without prior permission of the author.

Paperback ISBN: 9798822965997
eBook ISBN: 9798822966000

MY TESTIMONY

In the world, there are a large number of people who suffer on a daily basis from a number of things that happen in their daily lives; life in general is not easy, and we stumble through each day, trying to figure out how we can succeed and make it through that day. We all have a common goal to succeed in life and do well for our families no matter what the cost and hope we are teaching our children good values to live by. In my life, I saw good and terrible things as a child and all through my life, but I know that I made choices I thought were better for me at the moment. I was saved at the age of eight years, and I believed in God and Jesus Christ as my savior. I loved going to church and Sunday school, but as I got older, I placed other things that I thought were more important in front of God, like football, wrestling, and track. The other thing I placed in front of God was my determination to find someone to like me and go out with me, which made me feel kind of shallow when right in front of me was God and his son Jesus, who died for all the sins I committed in my life. All I had to do when I was younger was to give my all to God and let him guide me in my life, but as I would say to my dad when he would tell me things, "Things are different nowadays compared to when you were younger." But you know what? Times may be different, but the situations and choices you make are the same; they all have the same outcomes when you choose wrong. I found myself telling my kids that and receiving the same response that I gave my dad. The thing is, even if we were able now to go back in time and give ourselves better advice, we would never have the kids and family we have today. I understand some people would give anything to change their past, but God built me up with strength, patience, perseverance, humbleness, and forgiveness, and he was forgiving and showed me how to love again and forgive what others did to me. Those are things he helped me to develop over time. Even though I was hardheaded, he was there to carry me during those times. I thought I would just totally give up and let it go, not caring if I was missed but knowing that if I did end my life, no one would miss me, and everybody's lives would still go on. Those were hard times I went through and felt, because I hurt so much, and I wanted the pain to go away, but my biggest fear was if I took my life, God would send me to hell, and even when my son died, I prayed that God had taken him to heaven, where there was no more pain and suffering. After I wrote *Jordan's Voice*, a strong weight lifted from my shoulders, knowing I was letting the world know what I went through due to bullying and what Jordan went through due to bullying as well. I would have written the book years ago, but I would have placed a bigger target on myself in my job and would have been fired before I could have retired. I felt as I went along that I gave up on Jordan and that I failed him getting his word out as well as my story. I was cleaning out old work papers and college papers and found the notebooks that I had where I wrote my daily thoughts and what things I was going through. I then realized that I was retired and that I had the time and money to write our book and lift some of the doubts that I had in the past to write the story. I know that there are children and parents out there with a similar story who are afraid to step up and say something. Do not feel that way, and do not let the schools or people you work for make you feel helpless. I feel that every life matters, and if we do not step up and fight for our children or ourselves, then we have allowed those who bully us win without a fight. The thing is, it does not matter if you have never been bullied and you have never dealt with this behavior; your children have the right to go to school without fear of being harassed or bullied on a daily basis. I know firsthand how distracting being bullied was when I was in grade school; I could not focus on my learning, and it kept me from developing my learning skills and social skills. I know firsthand that in the workplace, harassment can affect your daily job performance, and your mind is not totally focused on your job, which becomes a problem for you and a safety issue as well. I remember a person telling me a long time ago that when you go to work, you leave home behind, and when you go home, you leave work behind. That is good advice, but many people have issues with leaving those things behind, and they come to work making other individuals live a nightmare while at work. The main problem, whether you are in school or a workplace: people hate the tattletale who goes and tells on what is going on and then makes their lives even more miserable than before. You are not being a tattletale; you are just wanting to be able to go to school or work in a stress-free environment and do your job the best that you can. Now, you may not believe in God, but I found after a long time of ignoring him, he was with me the whole time. I just needed to show him I had faith in his direction for me and to not give up, because he never gave up on me, and I thank him every day for the unconditional and eternal love he has given me.

I know that in life, people make fun of the way we look, talk, and dress, our heritage, who we think we are, and our beliefs, but that is not for someone else to decide or force upon us. I know as a Christian, there are things I do not agree on anymore compared to what I was around in life. Even when I knew who God was, I was not living on the path I should have been on. People would say you're not good enough, or they would never pick you or accept you; there is no use in trying to go that extra mile, because you do not matter. That was Satan telling me all that, and he was working through others to keep me from succeeding and being on that right path I was wanting to travel. There are a number of things I regret not fighting hard enough for in my life:

- Not allowing myself to have enough faith to allow God to handle my battles

- Not giving up and fighting harder for custody of my son

- Not giving up on my education, even though I had enough credits to earn my degree

- Not standing up sooner against the politics on my job, keeping myself from moving forward to allow me to become a better supervisor

- Not fighting hard enough to get a stronger bill passed for schools who do not enforce the guidelines for children who are bullied

- Taking too long to write mine and my son's story of bullying

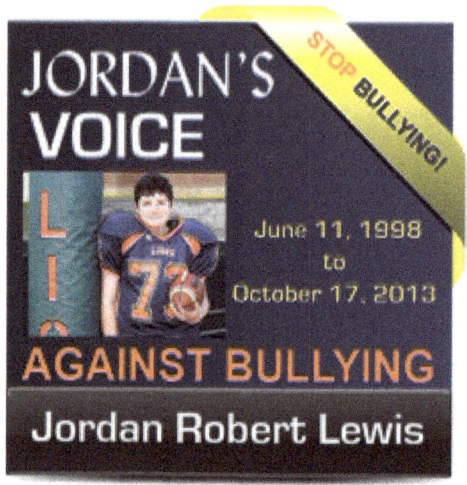

Thank you, dear Lord, for being there for me! Amen.
Bradley L. Lewis

CONTENTS

Author's Discussion ·1
Look through My Eyes· ·3
Chapter One ·6
Chapter Two ·13
Chapter Three ·21
Chapter Four ·29
Chapter Five· ·39
Chapter Six ·49
Chapter Seven ·59
Chapter Eight ·72
Chapter Nine ·83
Chapter Ten ·92
Chapter Eleven· 114
Chapter Twelve · 124

Wikipedia's definition of *bullying*:

> Bullying is the use of force, coercion, hurtful teasing, or threat to abuse, aggressively dominate or intimidate. The behavior is often repeated and habitual. One essential prerequisite is the perception (by the bully or by others) of an imbalance of physical or social power. This imbalance distinguishes bullying from conflict. Bullying is a subcategory of aggressive behavior characterized by hostile intent, imbalance of power and repetition over a period.

AUTHOR'S DISCUSSION

The concept of Jordan's Voice Against Bullying is for children to realize that their lives and their voices matter. Bullying takes place every day in this world, and many people say it is a concept we are never going to get rid of. Wrong! It can go away, but if you do not stand up against it, then it will not go away.

Children every day deal with bullying in so many ways in this generation; social media makes it harder for them to cope in their social environment at school without being made fun of and ridiculed for being different.

When we are younger, our skills are developed by our interaction with our families and our environment. Every family is different in how they interact with people, and we learn from that, but in addition to our parents teaching us, our environment and what we learn at school teach things. Every parent or household has different opinions on how to raise their children, so children's views on things tend to be different. As I stated, we learn from somewhere, and at times, we instruct our children on good or unhealthy habits; even though you may think they do not, children visualize your behavior as OK. So if we do not correct bad behaviors for children, children will carry those same bad behaviors into their lives if they are allowed to get by with them.

I grew up in a suburb of Chicago called Cicero, home of Italian mobster Al Capone, also known as Scarface. My parents were very protective of me growing up because they had lost a child three years prior due to drowning. I was also a hyperactive child. My family doctor refused to put me on meds because they could be addictive later in life. So from kindergarten through fifth grade, I was bullied, and believe me, it was not fun. Then from sixth grade to the beginning of eighth grade, I went to a Christian school, where I had no issues with bullying. My dad and mom divorced when I was in sixth grade, so when I started eighth grade, my dad asked if I wanted to move to Southern Illinois, and I said sure. I went through the rest of my schooling in the new town and never had to deal with bullying again.

I joined the active army, finished my time, and went back into society. When I got out, I stayed in the reserves and National Guard while I was searching for work. I thought that all the name-calling and harassment I endured in grade school was over, but I was wrong! Seven years later, I began working as a correctional officer for the state and spent twenty-six of my twenty-nine and a half years there being harassed, belittled, and restricted by management from training that would allow me to be promoted.

Now after all that time, I knew what the life of a roller coaster was like, but the worst of all of it was finding out my son was dealing with the same thing, and it caused him to take his life.

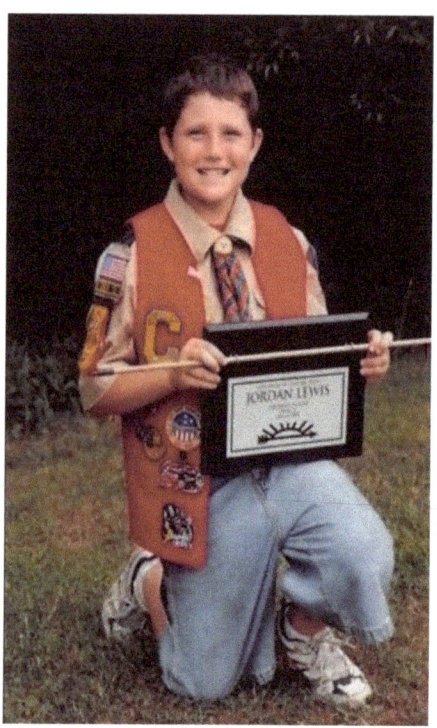

LOOK THROUGH MY EYES

How do you feel when you are watching a movie? What I mean is, when watching the movie, how does it make you feel? Do you imagine yourself as the character, feeling how that person is feeling during the highs and lows? Do you get caught up in the moment of the music and find yourself excited, happy, sad, frustrated, energized? And if it is a scary movie, do you feel goose bumps or your hair standing on end? Yes! Those are real feelings, because you can see how a person feels with the energy of the movie and music.

Now imagine a child going to school and being tormented from the time he sets foot on the bus headed to school until he sets foot on the bus coming home, or a child who walks to school in fear that someone will jump him out of nowhere. How do you think the child feels being made fun of for the way he looks or dresses, how he acts, his disability, the fact he is smart or his family is poor or he is sensitive? There are children who are so afraid of getting up in the morning and having to go to school that they pretend to be sick and skip school or become so sick inside they develop health problems or become so emotionally damaged that they cannot cope in a public setting. Many times, children are taken out of these environments and are homeschooled or placed in private schools for their safety and well-being. Imagine being in third grade and the kids pick on you, and when the teacher leaves the room, the kids throw things at you, like spitballs, eraser heads, or pieces of pencils broken apart. When the teacher comes back in, a few of the kids tell the teacher it was your fault. Then the teacher moves your desk to the corner by the door. The next time the teacher leaves, it starts again, and when she returns, there around your desk are pieces of paper, erasers, and pencils. The child looks up and

3

says, "See! I'm not doing anything." The teacher then replies, "I don't have enough corners to place them all in."

I remember when I was in first grade, I would get called on to answer a math question, but when I could not answer, the teacher would break my pencil. Every week, she would do it a couple of times, then one day I brought a whole handful of pencils to school. So when math class came, I waited till it was my turn. The teacher asked me, "What is the answer to this problem?" I did not know, and she thought I was being smart, but I was not. I was not particularly good in math at all, so she came up to me in front of my desk and said, "What is the answer?" and grabbed my pencil, beginning to bend it until it broke. I opened my desk and said, "That is OK—I have a bunch more."

She was mad and grabbed all my pencils and broke them. When school was over, she grabbed me by the arm and jerked me, walking fast out of the school door to go meet my mother. My mother was mad, and my sister, who is twelve years older than me, told her, "You let my brother alone, you witch."

What I am saying is, look through the eyes of your children, or if you are a student, the other kids around you. Try and see how afraid they may feel, because all they want to do is go to school and learn and make friends and even feel part of something as well. Karma is a good thing, but it also can be a terrible thing and come back and bite you in the butt. God said, "Do unto others as you would want them to do unto you." Both sayings mean the same thing, but God is karma, and he is about loving one another; when you hurt one of his children, his vengeance is the bad side of karma.

Right now, children do not see any farther than the nose in front of them. They feel invulnerable and feel that nothing can keep them from doing whatever they want. Children feel a lack of long-term consequences and think Mom and Dad can get them out of anything. Guess what? Sometimes they can, but the minute they cannot, you may be in a world of hurt, in a position where you may be locked up in jail for five, ten, or twenty years. I know because I work in corrections, and I have seen a few people I went to school with locked up because they thought that they were untouchable. Just ask three out of the four last governors in Illinois; they were on top, and no one could touch them.

Children and parents out there, please—I beg of you—take bullying seriously and help bring a law into effect on the federal level so that no other child must suffer and feel alone or isolated, so no other child feels their life has no meaning and that they are better off dead. Suicide is a one-way ticket, and there is no return trip, so take some time and project yourself into a child you are bullying at school, and just try and feel what they are feeling.

CHAPTER ONE

Where do you draw the line and say it is too much when joking with a person? You may be horseplaying, but does the other person consider it all fun and games? During my writing, I will try to discuss everything from my past to my present life, including what I have heard from other people, things I have endured, and some of what my son endured before taking his life due to bullying.

When looking back, I see I was a prayer answered by my parents. They had lost a son three years prior to me being born, due to drowning at Crab Orchard Lake during a family reunion. He was six years old, and his name was Roger Jr. Now he was survived by a brother, Phillip, who was three, and a sister, Linda, who was nine. The family was devastated by the loss. I remember stories; they would talk about how he was such a good boy, and my mother would say, "He was my little angel." The loss really hit my mother and sister hardest—not to say my dad did not feel anything. I know that when I was older, my mother did tell me that my father before he died said to her, "You really can't replace the ones you've lost." Then my parents carried a heavy heart, and both my parents prayed to God to deliver them another son, and three years later, God answered their prayers with me.

When I was growing up in the suburbs of Chicago, in Cicero, my parents were very overprotective of me, and I could have given them, to start, one good reason to be protective. When I was three years of age, we went to church, and on one Sunday, when I woke up, no one was up except my brother, who was catching the early bus for Sunday school. I asked him to take me since he was six years older than me, and he replied no. Everyone else was in bed, so I put my clothes on and went outside to water the flowers with the sprinkler can. While I was out there, the late bus drove up, and the driver asked me if I was going to church. Well, I said yes and headed into the house and took five silver dollars off my dad's dresser and went to church.

When Sunday school was over, I headed up to the main floor and saw my brother coming down the stairs. He asked me, "Who brought you?" I replied, "I rode the late bus to Sunday school." Well, that did not end there. As we walked outside the church, Mom and Dad pulled up, and yes, they were glad to see me, but after the hugs were given, the jail sentence came. Yeah, I was sentenced to play in the house or yard only. I did not have anyone my age nearby, so I spent a lot of time with GI Joe and Evel Knievel, and there was one specific time I gave my sister's Barbie dolls a haircut, which did not go over very well at all.

I remember my sister did a lot of babysitting, and there were times when my dad's sister would stay with us and watch me and my brother. The task was not that hard: keep an eye on the two boys. Well, it turned out that was a mistake by my parents. I was three years old at that time. My brother and I were outside playing; my brother would go up on the second-floor banister and slide down on it. My aunt called for my brother to come in, and my brother looked at me and said, "Stay off the banister." OK, you are telling a three-year-old who saw you do something fun no like it would sink in. Nope, I went up those stairs, and at the top, I climbed on that banister. I started to slide down, and that's when "Ah, shit" happened. I slipped off the banister and fell headfirst on the concrete. Screams were pouring out, then my aunt came running out.

Well, my mother called a little later to check in on us and asked my aunt how everything was. My aunt said, "Brad had a little fall and has a bump on his head." My mom, being overprotective as I mentioned, said, "What!" She dashed home from work, and when she saw my head, she lost it. I was rushed to our family doctor once my dad got home. Right away, my sister said, "If it were Halloween, you could dress up like Frankenstein's monster."

The doctor had to lance my forehead and drain the fluid off so he could stitch It up so it could heal, then three weeks later, I was running around the house and hit my head on my dad's knee, and I was Frankenstein's monster again.

Life was quite different after that for a while, up until I started kindergarten. At that point my life took a whole other direction, and I did not know how to deal with it. The first problem was, I did not know a single soul in my class; the second problem was that I knew nothing about how to socialize or talk to people. You know what is funny is that I can remember every classroom I have been in throughout my life and even my first bully in school (Joey). What was bad about him was he was two years older than the rest of the kids and big. There were these big red building blocks that we would make castles with, and he would run through, smashing them like he was Godzilla, but he looked like a big baby Huey. Now I would never say that aloud, fearing he could end my life with one punch. This was a period in which kids went to kindergarten all day and you brought a mat to school for nap time. When we went outside, it was at different times from the older kids so we would not get trampled on, and as school went by, it seemed to be all right except for Joey's presence every day. No one in school lived by me to see them. Plus, as a benefit, Mom always picked me up when school was over, and we went home so I could watch cartoons.

I remember Fridays were the time to get groceries, and no matter who I went with, when we went by the cereal aisle, it was quick, because they would put toys in that aisle, and if I saw something I wanted, I would cry for it. Well, both my parents had different tactics to deal with a screaming child. My mom would keep on walking into another aisle as if she did not know me; that would make me look like a total fool. On the other hand, my dad would jerk me up and bust my bottom right there in the store. Now, my dad made me hurt then, but Mom waited till I got home and placed me in a time-out and took television privileges away for a few days. The purpose was not to give in to me, and I know now that was a very acceptable thing, but it was not the last butt-busting I received. I realize now parents give in way too easily to their kids, and the kids learn no respect for their parents or others.

Jordan's Voice

Now, I do remember sometime during that year, I caught the back porch on fire, but do not start thinking I was a firebug either—I was like the little monkey called Curious George. My brother had these large matches on the back porch behind my sister's apartment; since she was working, she rented the apartment above our floor. There was a porch area where we played with my train and army men, plus we had hamsters up there that belonged to my sister and my brother. One day while my mom was lying down for a nap and my brother was in the living room watching television, I decided to go up the back stairs and play. I got hold of my brother's matches, striking them and watching them burn down, and when they would burn down to my fingers, I would flick them away so they would not burn my fingers. My brother called for me to come down and lie on the bed with Mom for a nap. I lay there for a bit, and after a short while, my mom started smelling something burning. She yelled for my brother to come to the room and said to him, "Go upstairs and see what is going on up there."

My brother ran up the stairs, and thirty seconds later, all I heard was my brother screaming through the door, "Mom, the house is on fire." My mom ran up the stairs and began beating on my sister's door to open it. They both pounded and screamed, then my sister finally opened her door. My mom burst into her apartment and filled buckets of water to throw on the back wall. A neighbor saw the smoke coming out the window and called the fire department. Before the fire department arrived, my mom, brother, and sister had put the fire out.

I was so scared. I was only five and a half years old, and I was begging my mom to whip me before Dad got home. I knew that this incident would spark severe rage in my dad's temper. Understand this: I deserved many whippings I received growing up, but I knew early in life, at this time, I was not ready for this whipping at all. You know, the scariest thing in a kid's life is not just God's wrath; it's also the wrath of the master of the house, which was my dad, and all I did was wait in my room till I heard the front door open. The thing is, I knew what the punishment was, and that was pain and suffering in a little kid's mind.

The front door opened. Dad was home. My mom met him at the front door, and I heard that sound of the belt being whipped off my dad's belt loops like it had oil on it. My dad would always say, "This is going to hurt me more than it will hurt you." Yeah, OK, as if I was supposed to believe that. When I became an adult and had to spank my kids with my hand, it hurt my hand, and it hurt my feelings to have to do that to my child. The thing is that emotional pain inside hurts a lot more than people think, and it stays with you for life, so when a child gets disciplined, you must remember it hurts a parent just as much to do the discipline. The reasoning behind it all is if a parent does not discipline their child, they show they do not care what happens to them in life, but there are rules to the degree of disciplining. There are times when you may think the child needs more, but you must restrain yourself and know you must implement other factors of disciplining. I look back and can say Mom and Dad gave me just the right amount of discipline, even though when I got older and looked back, I realized I might have deserved a little more.

Well, the whippings came and went along with the punishments, and I never played them ever again, but it did not take too long before I was in trouble for something else. You know I was restricted to the yard, but one day I saw my brother riding his ten-speed bike around the block, and I had to follow on my bike; it didn't go over very well when my mom came out and I wasn't in the yard. We were going around the block, and I thought it was cool following my brother until we pulled around to our house and my mother was on the front sidewalk, waiting. As soon as I pulled up to her, I was yanked off the bike and grounded for a week from television.

Summer was over, and it was time to start first grade. I was feeling like a big boy, and still, I did not have any friends in school. I had not seen anyone since kindergarten and felt awkward again. Now here is the kicker: I was a redheaded boy who wore black-framed glasses and had freckles everywhere; the glasses came because I scratched my retina so I could not see well out of my one eye. My life started out bad just because of my appearance alone, not accounting for being hyperactive, so when the kids began picking on me, it made it exceedingly difficult for me to focus on my learning. Now, you must remember, my brother was six years older than me, and my sister was twelve years older, so that left me with no one my age to play or socialize with. Then my parents wanted our doctor to prescribe medicine for my hyperactivity, but our doctor thought a lot about me and said, "No, I am not going to give this child medicine that could be addictive when he is older. He will grow out of it." Our doctor was good to us and had only the best intentions for me and knew that everything does not get fixed with a pill.

Our first-grade teacher was younger than most at the school, so I thought that would be a good thing. Yeah, right! School began, and yep, I was the main target to be made fun of, especially after the teacher pointed me out. This is where the bullying really began. I had trouble in math, so when the teacher would send me to the board to do a problem, I would really try, but I could not figure out the problem. The first month, the teacher targeted me. She would always come to me first and ask me for the answer to a problem on the board, and if I couldn't answer, she would grab my pencil and bend it, screaming at me, "Tell me the answer." Then, as I've mentioned, she would break the pencil. The kids in the class would laugh after she broke my pencil, and this would continue for weeks. I had to ask my mom to buy me new pencils. My mom was wondering why I needed new pencils so soon, but I said nothing, and one day I took a whole bundle of pencils to school wrapped in a rubber band. Well, it was math time, and the teacher came around to me and said, "What is the answer to the problem on the board?" I looked and tried figuring it out but could not complete it. Then she grabbed my pencil and began bending it in front of me, saying, "If you don't tell me the answer, I will break your pencil." I stated back to her, "I don't know it." Then she snapped my pencil.

Well, I felt like I had to step up and stand up to her, so I reached into my desk and pulled out my bundle of pencils wrapped with a rubber band. I then stated, "That's OK; I have all these other pencils." The kids began to laugh. She grabbed the whole bunch out of my hand and tried breaking them all at once. The kids began to laugh more, so she broke each one individually; the kids still laughed at her. Then she told me I had to stay after school. After all the kids left, she walked me out, jerking me by the arm to my mom's car, but my sister, who was twelve years older than me, told her, "You get your hands off my brother, you witch." My eyes got big, and I thought my sister had said the b-word. In my mind, I thought, wow, my sister stepped up and took the blame off me, and she is mad,wow mom then stepped in and made statements that would have erupted into a fight, but my mom instead went to the principal's office. She related what had happened and everything else the teacher was doing to me in class.

Well, the pencil breaking stopped, but the teacher started doing something that continued for a long time to come. During lunch period, kids would chase me all around the playground, and when I had to walk home after school, they would chase me down and punch or shove me to the ground. I would sometimes run to the front door of a house and ring the doorbell until someone answered. Then that person would chase the kids away, but sometimes they told me to get off their porch. I had to figure out new ways to get away from them and make it home safely. There were times I would run to the back of a house and hide in a basement crawl space or run into yards and begin jumping over fences to get away. Honestly, some of those tactics worked, but many failed, because I would get chased away by the owners, and if I told Mom, then I would not be able to walk to school or home by myself either. I found that when going to school, I would have to change my routes, because the bullies would be waiting for me, and I would have to wait until the school bell rang to get in while at the same time avoiding being tardy.

CHAPTER TWO

Second grade was the same, and I found it hard at times to focus on what the teacher was saying because I was plotting my escape route from the bullies on the playground and then my route after school until I reached the gate and made it into my yard. I remember a time in second grade when we had free time to play in the classroom. Two other kids and I were playing with pick-up sticks under a table. A boy named Brian barged in and said he was playing. I said to him we already started and he would have to wait till we finished. Brian did not want to hear that, so he shoved a wooden chair back against the table, then he kicked it back farther, so hard it slammed into my forehead and left a huge goose egg. Remember the couple of forehead injuries I had when I was younger? My mom freaked out when she had to come to school and pick me up. Now, the kid got in trouble for what he did. No, there was not a suspension; they had his parents come in and agreed on a week of no recess on the playground.

Aside from being bullied, I did enjoy school and wanted to be part of something and try to interact, but same old thing—I was not allowed over to anyone's house. Third grade came, and it was another year of excitement, the same routine, just a little more physical and new creative names like "red on the head like a pecker on a poodle" or "freckle-face four eyes."

I will share an incident with you that has never gone away in my mind. I was in third grade, and when the teacher would leave the room, the bullies would start throwing things at me. When the teacher came in and said, "What is all the commotion going on?" the fingers pointed at me, so I was placed in the corner by the door. Then when the teacher would walk out, I would get bombarded by spit wads, eraser heads, and pieces of pencils. Then when she came back into the classroom and looked around my desk, I would look at her and say, "See, they are doing it," and the response I would receive, as I've already told you, was, "There are not enough corners to place them in." My head dropped, and I felt this would never work for me.

Back at this time in my life, there was no such thing as kids committing suicide, but I would find myself crying somewhere alone, wishing I had never been born and that I were dead. I never had any tendencies to hurt myself. Why? Because I was getting enough pain physically and emotionally at school from the other kids, so why hurt myself?

The family was going to church during these years, and I had friends at church and went to church activities, but none of the kids lived near me or went to my school, so just seeing them once a week on Sundays and a few hours on Wednesday night really didn't add up to much. Still, I prayed to God to help me or to take me away from this life. I felt that in the radius of four blocks in three directions from school to my house, people knew the little redheaded kid with freckles and glasses ringing their doorbells or running into their stores and hiding from the kids. I would go out of my way and run out the back door of the school at times to change my routine to avoid the group waiting for me. I had to try and make it quick, because Mom knew how long it took me to walk home every day, and she would allow a five- to ten-minute window, and if I was not there, she would come looking for me.

My dad worked a lot and took care of the house and vehicle; my mom worked, cooked, cleaned the house, and managed the bills. We had a noticeably big backyard, which was not common in Cicero, but we were also one block from being in Chicago, so I did have plenty of play space for myself. I was never a child who made imaginary friends when I was younger, so I had no friends at all, just acquaintances from church. There were times in the schoolyard when I couldn't get away from the kids, and I would climb a ten-foot fence to get over and away from them, but that did not work since they would run around in the alley and head me off on the other side. This was a daily routine unless someone else came around and did something stupid that would take the blame off me.

Jordan's Voice

Fourth grade came, and I was in Ms. Finkle's class. She had been one of my brother's teachers, and she knew already that I was not like my brother. We also started dressing out for physical education class and had to wear a jock under our shorts and shower after. There was an incident during the first part of the school year where a kid named Freddy, whom I had to share my locker with, decided one day to take my clean pair of underwear and leave me with his. I said something to the gym coach, and he asked Freddy if he was wearing my underwear. Freddy played the game and got a couple other boys to agree with him, so the coach told me to wear the other underwear, which had urine stains and a brown streak on it. I was upset; I did not want to wear someone else's poopy underwear, but the coach made me. Then they called me poopy pants. I really did not need that after all the other things. I mean, instead of putting me in the corner, I was moved to the hallway at times.

I went home and told my mom, and she was mad and contacted Freddy's mother. The next day, my mom put the underwear in a plastic bag for me to drop off at his house on the way to school, at which point, I would also pick up mine. The mother didn't even apologize at all. The next day I went to school, and I showed the gym coach my underwear after dressing out and said, "See, these are mine. They do not have the same waistband color as his." Same response as Freddy's mom—no apology for his mistake.

Sometime midway through the school year, we moved across town in Cicero. I continued my fourth-grade year at McKinnley School. This school only went to fourth grade, then in fifth grade, students would transfer to Burnham School. I was excited and scared. How would I deal with this school? All I wanted to do was make friends and be liked by the other kids. Well, my first day, the guys were glad, because it meant there were more boys than girls, and they wanted to outnumber the girls on votes when deciding on extra special things in class. That was all good and everything was going well until I developed a crush on this girl in class named Sandy and came to find out after talking to her that the biggest and toughest boy also liked her. He looked like a badass, like a young Charles Bronson without the mustache, and he even had a scar on his cheek. Wow! Why did this have to happen? The names and chasing me to and from school started all over, because he was making it his mission to make my life hell. There were fewer options now; in fact, there were no options at all. The teacher would let me leave three minutes before the bell rang to give me a head start getting home. There was a lot of dogging and having to run faster at times, but now, since I was in fourth grade, the punches hurt a lot more.

The problem with bullying for me was it affected my grades, plus it was not easy watching the toughest guy in school look at me and remind me what was coming when the bell rang. Sometimes you would think these guys had something to do, like hobbies to occupy their time, but no, tormenting me every day was their hobby.

I did know some neighbor boys who were four years older than me and lived a couple houses down and went to church with us, but they were at Burnham. When they were not busy, they would come over and play board games, or we would shoot basketball in the alley behind their garage. Our church needed a bigger space, so they bought the church across from my school, which made it easier to walk to church for me and my brother; my sister did not go anymore, so it was my mom, dad, and brother. Church was my haven on Sundays, but since I walked to and from church, I had to look out for the kids I went to school with roaming the neighborhood in case I had to make a quick dash and run for my life.

I would find things to do at times. For instance, when my dad went to the grocery store, I would go with him, because there was money to be made helping people get their bags out of the cart and putting them in their cars. I would make twenty-five cents to a dollar as a tip depending on how generous the people were, and in one hour, I could make twenty dollars or more depending on how fast I hustled. One day my dad asked me if I had stolen the money, and I said no, then I had my dad stand by his car and watch me make the money. My dad was surprised and proud of me that I had made the effort to earn my own money, but when my brother borrowed money and didn't pay it back, Dad would pay me back and tell me if he needed money, he could earn it like I did. I earned money with different jobs, like mowing yards, shoveling snow, or even pulling nails out of boards; I would get a nickel for small nails and a dime for big nails.

In the previous three years, we had not gone on vacation, so Dad picked up a summer pass for the local pool, and I would go every chance I could. I did not have to worry about kids picking on me there because of the lifeguards, and it was only a block from my house, which meant I did not have to run far to get home.

The start of my fifth-grade year was different. As I mentioned, everyone who was at McKinnley School for fourth grade had to go to Burnham for fifth to eighth grade, which meant a bigger school and four to five fifth-grade classes; there were thus more kids than usual to pick on me. My dad decided to sign me up for Little League football, which was part of the park district, and practice was every day after school. The team was made up of kids from fifth grade to sixth grade. We had enough kids to make two teams, and we practiced together during the week. I liked the idea of playing because it gave me an opportunity to take my anger out on the field, even though I was skinny for my size. I was not a good football player, but I went out and did my best because I wanted to be a part of something bigger, because I wanted to feel useful and feel as if I belonged as a part of something. I know there are other kids going through the same thing around the world that I was then, but when you are young, you feel all alone and separated as an outcast from society.

Well, as I stated earlier, a bigger school meant more kids, and still, I could not focus, plus the candy I would buy before school at the dime store did not help my hyperactivity; I would reach into my desk and eat it during class. Between waiting a block away before school or running off school grounds during lunch to hide until the bell rang and hurrying back in, I had to improvise to survive, even when the teacher would let me leave three minutes before the bell rang to give me a head start to run home. She would tell me to run straight home, and I would, then while running, I would hear that bell ring; I would look back to see if anyone was behind me chasing me. Sometimes they would not follow me, but if they did, I would kick it up and run a little faster, because I had to get home. I also had to get something to drink and get dressed for football practice.

Now, on the practice field, it was one-on-one, and I would try and take my aggressions out against the ones who picked on me; even though sometimes they would double-team me, I would still push through them with all my might. After practice, everyone was usually too tired to try and bother me, which was a relief, because I was tired and I had to go home and do my homework, a priority after showering. Playing Park district Little League football kept me busy, but still, I always had that time at school when the handful of boys would continue to torment me.

I remember the year prior, my dad rented out the basement flat to a woman and her daughter. After about four months, there was arguing coming from the house, plus food was in the windows since it was cold, and we found food in the snow in the gangway between the houses. The woman then got behind on rent for four months, and my dad had to evict them; the police came and had their things placed out by the curb because they refused the eviction order. The reason I'm mentioning this is that a month later, the daughter, who was three years older than me and went to my school and was bigger, had a couple of friends in eighth grade corner me and beat me up on a porch across from school, off school grounds. Her friends held me, and she pulled my hair and hit me, saying, "You and your family kicked us out on the streets, and you helped carry stuff out, so I am going to beat your ass." Luckily, the lady who owned the house came out and chased them away, but she said she was not done with me yet. Every day for the rest of the school year, I would look for her. Even though my parents went to the principal's office and complained to him, his reply was, "If it happened before or after school, off school grounds, we can't do anything about it."

Well, my grades were suffering, and the teacher put my desk in the clothes closet in the back or in the hallway, which made it hard for me to hear her or ask questions about something I did not know. The sad thing for me was it was the end of the school year, and I was expecting to be held back because of my grades. The teacher started handing the report cards out, and when she gave me mine, I opened it and looked. My stomach dropped. I did not fail, but how I did not was unknown to me. I had nine Ds and one U. I knew my parents were going to become truly angry.

We all lined up at the door to leave to go home, and as usual, the teacher let me leave three minutes early to have time to get home. When she opened the door, I dashed right out and ran. I was not going to look back, because for one, I was thinking of how bad my rear end was going to feel when Dad got ahold of me. I was at least five blocks away from school, and out of nowhere, I was grabbed and pulled into the alley. There were four eighth-grade boys surrounding me; one was a friend of the girl who lived in our basement—she was there as well—and the other three were brothers of kids in my class, so there were five total. They were out earlier than the rest of us because they were going to high school next year, so they waited for me on the route I usually ran to go home. They took their turns at me, and I was hurting; my lip was split, and I knew I was bruised as well. When they were through, they left me alone. I got up slowly after they left and headed home. I knew this was a godsend for me, because my parents would have pity on me, and I would not get the butt-whipping of a lifetime.

I arrived home, and when they got home from work, they were all outraged at the way I looked; I had a busted lip, abrasions on my forehead, scrapes on my arms, and black eyes. I gave my parents the report card, but they did not care what was on it; I passed, and they were more concerned about my condition. This was the first time getting beaten up was a lot better than my dad whipping me and grounding me for the summer. Now, my mom and dad gave me a good lecture, but as I told them, when I did not understand something, I would ask questions, and then the kids would say that I was distracting them. I told them that when I told the teacher I did not understand, my desk was moved into the hall, so I was not able to learn much. That was why I was not learning.

So, in this example, overall, the victim is punished and loses out on trying to learn and be educated, so they become less motivated and want to make less of an effort. Besides the lack of motivation, they become more isolated through this manner of behavioral treatment by teachers; kids really do not want to have anything to do with them because they are the outsider of the class, and so making friends becomes less of an option. Now, how does this type of behavior affect a child? Are there other outside factors? In my situation, my mom and dad disciplined me when I needed it and did not abuse me. My mom and dad were very protective of me and did not let us run wild but made sure we knew what was right and wrong. Do we as kids always do what we are told? No. We have moments when we lie or steal some candy or pocket change, for example. There are times we break things and do not say anything. But my mom and dad would discipline us if we were caught. So no, my mom and dad would never condone me, my brother, or my sister bullying other kids; instead, there would be a butt-whipping coming.

Now, I am not going to make my parents appear to be angels, but my mom and dad were good people. Dad, when I was younger, would drink, and he and my mom would argue at times and then go to bed. When Dad did drink, he was not a violent person; he was a happy drinker who would hug people and kiss people. It was annoying and embarrassing to my mom, but Dad quit drinking after getting robbed twice. The main thing I knew about my parents was that they did have values and never lived beyond their means. My dad dropped out of school after sixth grade to work on the farm and deliver coal to help the family. My mom went to school up till ninth grade, and she met my dad after he came back home from the Korean War. Both were very diligent workers and were never in debt.

When people look at a child now who has been bullied or—let us go on this route—when a child commits suicide and this child was bullied, people or the community want to say the child had a poor home life. I never thought of committing suicide; yes, I might have prayed to God and wished I were dead or had never been born, but I feared God and feared I would go to hell if I did. I did cry and wonder, Why take Roger Jr. and replace him with me? Those were thoughts I had often, and I wished things were different.

CHAPTER THREE

The following year was sixth grade, and my dad enrolled me in a Christian school out in Oak Forest. I would ride with a lady from church and her five kids and a couple of others from church. Now this was different, because we wore uniforms, and the teachers were able to paddle you on your butt. This was a new concept, and I learned fast how you got paddled: three demerits get you one paddle in one day, and six, you receive two paddling's. Now, that was for a day. At the end of each semester, if you had accumulated ten demerits, it was one paddling; twenty was two paddlings; thirty was three paddlings; and so on. I received paddlings during the semester, and I earned four paddlings at the end of my first semester, but after that, I learned getting hit on the butt with a wooden paddle with holes hurts more than a leather belt. I did get paddled again, but the second semester was two paddlings, and the third and fourth semester, I received only one.

I was not bullied, my grades went up significantly, and as for friends, the school was twenty miles away, so I mostly had acquaintances. The only friends I did have were the two boys next door, Sam and Dan, twins; we would play basketball in the alley or at the church, and we all went to church on Wednesday and Sunday. We had church activities: I played on the church basketball team and softball team, and it was a lot better than dealing with kids in the public schools. You may think I am joking, but living on the edge of Chicago, kids wanted to make names for themselves before high school. The Christian school was completely different; it was about getting along and teaching better values.

Now that spring had arrived, I was playing softball in a deserted lot down from the church. The ball went into the busy street, and I ran across, looking for traffic; when I picked the ball up and turned to recross the street, I was hit by a car. The youth pastor and my dad came running. I was down and saw stars when my head hit the concrete. The person that hit me was a fifteen-year-old driving with his dad, and he rushed to make the turn signal to turn left. The ambulance came, and I was rushed to the hospital. My dad drove with us. When we arrived, they took X-rays and found I had a broken tibia. The doctor placed a cast with a walking heel, and I was taken upstairs for overnight observation.

My mom got to the hospital; my dad was still there with me. After talking to me for a while, they said they had something to discuss with me. I said, "OK." Mom looked at me and said, "Me and your dad are separating and getting a divorce from each other." I really did not know what to say! I asked why and for what reason, and all they could say was things changed and they grew apart, but I found out later my mom had had an affair and met another man at her work. My mom and dad were sensible about custody and asked who I wanted to live with. I said, "Dad." The reason was, I did not want to move and have to go back to a public school; I was content where I was and had my own room.

The school year ended. The summer was time for me to go swimming, and Dad let me walk to the movies on my own; that was important to me—being able to walk eight blocks with the money I earned carrying groceries. I remember I went to see *H.O.T.S.* It was a college movie like *Animal House* and was rated R. I am not going to say anything to anyone except it was great, and I enjoyed my independence.

I was finished with grade school and entered junior high. I also gained a part-time job during the summer, working for a gentleman from church who owned five restaurants, one of which was within riding distance for me on my ten-speed bike. The place was five miles from where I lived and was down by Sportsman Park, by all the trucking hubs. I got up early on Saturdays and during the week and worked five hours each day except Sunday, and the manager paid me in cash after each day. I washed dishes and put stock away and cleaned tables off, sweeping and mopping; it kept me busy, and I made money doing things, and that made me feel good about myself. I did this for most of the summer, and during this time, my brother moved in with my mom so he could be closer to his girlfriend's house. I knew he would try and ask me for money, but since he did not have a job that would allow him to pay me back, it was not going to happen. I learned my lesson from a few years back, when my dad had to pay me the money back.

I didn't think that my mom and dad getting divorced was the reason for my increased freedom. It's just my dad realized I needed to grow up and become responsible; there was much to learn about, and I didn't even have a clue yet. My dad and I drove out to Wichita, Kansas, where my uncle lived; he was my dad's youngest brother. The drive from Chicago was exceptionally long, and when you hopped onto a turnpike, if you had to use the bathroom or get something to eat or drink, then you were going to wait a while. We arrived and met my uncle and his new wife and children. They were genuinely nice people. We even took a ride to Silver Dollar City, which is just across the state line in Missouri. We spent half the day there and then drove back to my uncle's house.

We stayed for a week, then headed back home. My dad was enrolling me at another Christian school, because the lady at our church was not taking her kids back there because of the cost and her being a single mother. This school had a bus that drove to the area and picked up the kids, so here was another school and a new experience. The school year had begun. The ride to school and home took a while due to the city traffic on the expressway, but there were a few kids that lived close by and others who were about five blocks away. A boy named Kenny and his sister lived six houses down on the opposite side of the street. We became friends, and that year, I joined the school basketball team. It was fun, even though I was not particularly good at it. The classes were quite different from the other Christian school because the other school operated according to individual paces, as they called it—when you finished a section on your own, you went to the next at your own pace. The school science class worked with chemicals and allowed you to do experiments using Bunsen burners and make things like batteries from scratch. It was hard to like a girl because they all lived in other towns, but there was one I would talk to on the phone sometimes; that was the extent of me having a girlfriend in seventh grade.

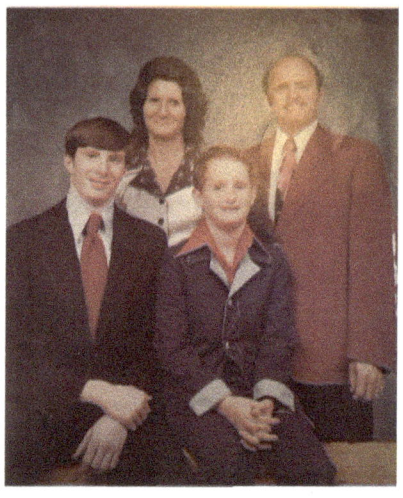

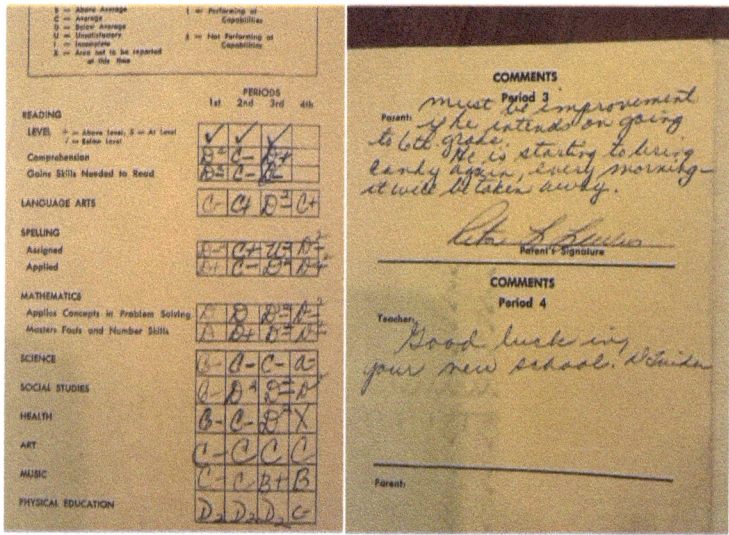

This was what I looked like in fifth grade, and these were my grades throughout the year due to being bullied and not being able to focus on the classroom the way a child should be able to.

About three-quarters of the way through the school year, my dad had a heart attack at work, and eventually, he could not go back to work in the factory. My dad worked as a crane operator, and the heat in the factory was extreme up top. I had experienced two full years of no bullying or being beaten up, but my dad decided that since he was being placed on social security disability, we should move down south to Marion, where he grew up. I really had no problem with that, because starting in my eighth-grade year, I had to go back to public school and deal with the same old crowd again. I could not imagine dealing with this group of kids again; even though I had been away for a couple of years, I knew they were not going to forget me.

My dad had found a trailer out by the Lake of Egypt and borrowed money from my bank account, which was funded with money I received from the lawsuit when I was hit by a car and child support money my mom had given to me so he could purchase the trailer. I had to start the first two weeks of my eighth-grade year at Burnham School in Cicero. As I had thought, a few kids remembered me and started chasing me after school, but I just waited my time out till the two weeks were over. We headed out on Friday, leaving with our personal belongings and a small trailer of furniture to put in the trailer. I hated moving, but sometimes you do not have complete control over everything when others are involved.

The first day, I waited at the bus stop for the bus, having had to get up early because we lived ten miles out of town and the bus came early; with all the stops, the ride was forty-five minutes long. When I arrived at school, I went to my locker to make sure I knew my combination, put my backpack away, and look over my class schedule to figure out where each class was. The atmosphere was different in some ways, and I even started liking the kids; they were a little more friendly, but I was going from a city environment to a country environment, so behaviors were quite different. I tried going out for basketball, but that was a disappointment right away. Some guys started showing off during drills, making me look bad, which I was—I will not argue with that! So I never went back to practice, knowing where I stood. I made friends, especially with kids who lived near me, and found out that a third cousin lived just down the road from me and was in the same grade. It was fun living out by the lake at times. I would go fishing, and one of my dad's cousins gave us a German shepherd so I would have someone to run around with at the lake. My dog's name was Smokey, and he was my best friend, running everywhere I went; he would swim across a cove of the lake to get to another friend's house. He was my protector, and in the fall and winter, we would walk out in the woods and sit back under a fir tree with the snow encapsulating the tree in a dry, warm area underneath, out from the wind, and just relax. I would lay there talking to him, even though he could not answer me; he would just lie there next to me and listen. I found that being out in a secluded area by the lake was very soothing for me.

Now, on the weekends, Dad would drive me into town and drop me off around five in the evening at the movies so I could watch the early show and the regular show, then would pick me up at the pizza place across the street from the movies. This was a routine every Friday night, even when I had a friend stay over; we would head into town and watch movies until my dad was finished at the Elks club. Saturdays, I would get up early, then go fishing most of the day. Smokey, my dog, would go with me and would have a blast chasing rabbits and playing in the water down by the spillway. He would provide added entertainment while I fished, and it made time go by as well.

I decided that spring to go out for track, because during gym class, we were timed while running around the track, and the gym coach suggested that I should go out for the mile in track. I figured, why not? My brother ran long distance in high school, and he was good at it, so I agreed. We started with the field events; I tried high jumping. I did good, but then they called us for preparation for the mile. I was nervous, as this was my first track meet. I went over close to where we were supposed to start the race, and I stretched out my legs good, then they called us up to get on the track and line up in our positions. I was nervous, and my heart was pounding. They said, "Get on your marks! Get set!" and the gun went off. I took off. All I had in my mind was the instinct to run as fast as I could and not look back till I reached home. That was the memory in my mind from living in Cicero; I felt like kids were chasing me again to beat me up. This was not a feeling I wanted to feel, but it was the first thing that came into my mind when I took off running. I had never learned how to run long distance—it was more of a fight-or-flight scenario when I was younger—so I paced myself and reserved just enough for the end and gave it all I had to finish. When I made it to the finish line, the timekeeper approached me with my time and said, "Son, you broke the eighth-grade record, running a 5:49 mile." The previous record was 5:55, and I had shattered it. Running a 5:49 mile my first time, I was excited and continued running the mile event and competing in high jump as well.

The season went on, and I kept on breaking the record, until at state, I got third place and ran a 5:09 mile; I was happy, and everyone else was happy for me. That is when things really changed for me. I got along great with everyone and had friends, but I did not have a girlfriend. In fact, over the previous years, a lot had changed for me, like not having to wear glasses anymore and growing taller. I did not appeal to many girls. Why, I really could not say, beyond my looks and my inability to socialize well. I mean, you can be the sweetest guy, but if you do not have an appeal, then your chances are slim. I was insecure—with being pushed, shoved, and beat up, how you would expect me to feel beyond awkward? I had no real personality, and how was I supposed to develop one? I wanted to be friends with everyone. I was decent in sports, and people noticed me, but I would always hear, "He is just a sweetheart." I wanted to be wanted and loved—nothing sexual, only deep feelings and caring. I had a lot of emotions as a child and I felt for others, but I carried my emotions on my sleeve and got hurt. That may have been a reason I was picked on as well, but even though I thought I was the only one like this, I was wrong! I learned later in life that I knew someone else just like me.

Eighth grade was over, and now, I was a big first-year student and a little fish in a bigger pond again. I played football for two years, wrestled for four years, and ran track for three years; the only reason it wasn't four was I got hurt in wrestling my senior year. I played second-string defense, which tells you I was not a big player, and I was also the kicker who kicked the ball off. Besides that, I did not have much of a football career. I did enjoy wrestling because it was a one-on-one sport and, in a way, something through which I could take out aggression as well; I started out my freshman year only losing one match and being overweight at the conference tournament. The coach was mad. I should not have had that pizza the night before, even though it was just two slices. I did wrestle conference my sophomore year and took second or third. My junior year, I did not wrestle as much, because I had to wrestle a senior in my weight class, who was good until he got hurt; I finished the rest of the year. My senior year, I wrestled just a part of the season until I tore a ligament in my left knee, which ended my season for wrestling and track.

I ran track for three years, running the eight-hundred-meter relay and the mile. Now, there was a guy two years older than me named Scott, and he became a friend of mine. Scott was a good runner; he was my competition, but he was the one who pushed me harder, and during those first two years, we had a blast. I continued my junior year, and I ran well that year, except for regionals. I paced the guy from Benton to break the regional record, and I burned out on the last lap on the back straightaway. Now, I had my fastest time that year, and it was 4:32; that was four seconds from the school record. Was I pissed about not running my senior year? Yeah, but I had already enlisted in the army at the beginning of the school year on a delay entry program, so I had to heal.

CHAPTER FOUR

Graduation was over, and I was heading off for a new adventure in the United States Army. I enlisted another friend of mine, whose name was Scott; I graduated with him, and we signed up together in the same field. I originally tried for topographic engineer, but that was all filled, so it was artillery surveyor 82C. The one thing that was different between me and my friend was he signed up for a three-year enlistment, and I took the two-year, which was just offered. When I received my duty station during AIT, which is training in the job we enlisted to do, field artillery surveyor Scott received his as well, and he was not happy. I was assigned Fort Campbell, Kentucky, and he was assigned South Korea, a one-year, hard-duty tour on which you could not take family with you if you had any.

The end of my two years finally came, and a sergeant major wanted me to enlist in a special forces group that was just being set up and taking interviews. I had to decline, because I wanted to get out and start my life, but I did go into the reserves and National Guard. I took a job as a teacher's assistant in special education, where I worked as a one-on-one aide for a special needs child. I worked about two years doing this, and I met my first wife in town during this time. The job was very stressful, even more than the physical things we did in the army, and doing this kind of work allows you to understand how lucky you are, at the same time, your heart hurts for these children. I watched kids make fun of how these children looked, talked, or walked, and I realized that these kids could get away either, and I would say something to them; it would stop for a while and happen again at a different time. The child I was assigned to was bound to a wheelchair and was dependent on me to take him to the bathroom and feed him; he could not talk and had a word board that was attached to his wheelchair like a table on which he could point to words and pictures.

I married my wife a year and a half after we met because she was pregnant, and I felt I should do the right thing. My mom told me I did not have to marry her and could still support the child. Now, on the other hand, my dad was telling me there was only one thing to do, and that was get married, since I was still living with him. Here I was feeling confused, thinking I wanted to be with someone who accepted me and realized I was a good person, but even her father warned me she was not ready to be in a relationship, because she had more issues she needed to deal with.

Life is not simple, but a person should be able to go through life knowing that if they try and work hard and are good to others, they should be treated well; that, people say, is wishful thinking and something you could only hope for. I was searching for the realization that the right person was out there for me, but was I being patient enough, or was I searching too hard? While I was growing up, I would watch movies, especially at the theater. It was an escape from reality for me, imagining I was the person on the big screen, a different person with a different life.

My wife and I were married just shy of five years, and we had a daughter; her name is Deeanna. I worked two jobs at this time to pay the bills—I worked for my family doctor during the morning and then at the factory in the evening. When I was at my doctor's house, I would do repairs and paint, and there were times on the weekend I worked on his lake house. At night, I worked the factory where my mother and her second husband worked. I would put in full shifts, and if there was overtime, I would take it and give myself about four or five hours of sleep every night. That was the big reason my wife and I divorced—I was working all the time, and she was fooling around.

I finally found a solid job working for corrections as a correctional officer. The only problem was, the first day at the academy was my divorce date, and I had to make a choice: a good-paying job to take care of my kids or fighting for custody with no job. I went to the academy, and she received custody of the children. Now, for the first six to seven weeks, I was busy at the academy. I found a little trailer to live in until I could get money saved back so I could move somewhere better where my kids could stay.

After the academy was over, we went back to our institutions, and the first week consisted of becoming informed about how our institution was run and forgetting about everything we learned at the academy, because they did things differently. This was different, but if I was going to get along, I needed to adhere to what I was told. My first assignment was in the west building, and I was assigned to a senior officer to shadow him for the day. I followed and watched him get inmates out of their cells and observed how count was performed; three hours in, the officer handed me the keys and said, "You are on your own." I went ahead and did everything the way he did and even went to cells to get inmates out for their call passes to the health care center, school, and library.

The first day was different; the cell house was filled with smoke from all the inmates and staff smoking, then the noise was crazy, with inmates' televisions on in their cells and yelling to one another in their cells. I went home that night and tried to piece together my first day. I was nervous in this unfamiliar environment, where there were five hundred inmates in a cell house, and they were in prison for murder, rape, assault, drugs, child molestation, and so on. I sat in my recliner and thought about the fact that I was there because it was a full-time job with great health benefits and good pay, and that was what I had to do to take care of my children.

I worked for about three months, then I started waking up in the middle of the night imagining I was locked up and the officers I worked with were my gallery officers. I would be dripping in sweat, cool and clammy all over. So I decided I was going to go to college and get my degree as a counselor so I could do something better than what I was doing there. The reason I decided to go to school was not the inmates altogether but the staff I worked with daily, who made me feel like I was back in grade school. The pranks, the harassment—putting a lit cigarette in your pocket, placing ink on the phone receiver, stapling the arms of your jacket closed and putting cups of water in the sleeve—and if you said something, they would twist it all around and make you look like a dumbass.

So that summer, I signed up at the junior college and took a psychology class just to give myself a feel for whether I would like college, and I ended up getting a B-plus in the class; I went ahead and signed up for three more classes in the fall semester. I was busy every day, with three classes in the morning, heading to work after school, picking up something on the way there to eat for my lunch, going through the chaotic rituals of work for eight hours, then coming home for six hours of sleep and getting back up for the same routine. I was at the end of my third semester, and I was taking three classes a semester and a couple of summer classes to get things rolling and to keep my mind off work and the daily harassment I was dealing with.

I started going out and seeing if I could meet someone, but things were hard. I saw this local article, and I replied to it. The woman sounded sincere, and when she called, she did not sound so bad, so we met at the local bar. I was living in a three-bedroom apartment, and the bar was just a block from my house. When I met her, I saw she was a nice-looking woman. As we talked, I learned she was starting her fourth semester at the junior college I went to. In my mind, I thought, here is a person motivated to earn her degree and do something with herself, so we dated for a while. After a while, she seemed concerned about my kids and how they were living, and I was glad she felt that way. We talked, and I decided to take custody of my two children. She did not have a problem, so we got engaged to make it more likely I would get custody, since she was living with me. I talked to my lawyer; since my ex-wife had moved about four times in three years and my son had gotten held back a grade from missing too many days of school, I was rewarded with primary custody, and they lived with me.

We were married by the end of my third year in junior college. She was finishing her associate's degree, and she started getting overwhelmed dealing with the kids at night, so we talked about me going to a day shift. The problem with that was, I had to switch my classes to one day a week, so I transferred to the main college and took four classes a day. That allowed me to be home after work and take care of my kids, and I would do my homework at night and study. I started seeing a lot of behavioral changes in my wife and how she treated my kids—yelling at them and jerking them around to make them behave—so unexpectedly, I told her, "If you can't deal with the kids properly, you can pack your things and leave." She couldn't believe I said that and replied, "You would kick me out over the kids?" and I replied, "Yes." I wasn't going to deal with them being treated badly. That's when she said, "I'm feeling left out; my friends are pregnant and having babies, and I don't have one of my own."

I had to think about it hard. I mean, I was getting harassed after one incident. She didn't come home one night after being out with a girlfriend down in Paducah. I said something to my shift commander, asking if I could go back home to see where she was and if everything was all right. That's when guys in the cell house started saying, "Was that you calling? I took that pager, tapped it to her ass, and was whaling away on that ass." I was mad and went into the bathroom, pounding on the door with my hand then splashing water in my face. One of our big guards, Bob, pulled the door open and said, "Son, you don't have to beat your head in the door," and from that day on, for a good six months, when I went to the bathroom, they would have a sponge stapled to the door with a paper saying, "In case of an emergency, pound your head here." So it was hard for me at home and at work, and the only thing I could do was decompress, going to work, going home, and then sinking my head into my books, studying.

Remember I said that I would go to the movies and forget about the world and imagine I was a character in the movie? I would do that after my last class on Wednesday nights before I went home. That was the only way for me to escape reality and keep my sanity—to sit back and place myself in the movie. I mean, I had plenty of moments talking to God on my drives to and from work, asking him for direction.

I then talked to my wife about having a baby and how things might change between us. So we got pregnant, and we had a baby boy. I named him Jordan, and she decided his middle name would be her dad's name, Robert. Now, I don't know why she named him after her dad; when we were dating, she wrote me a three-page letter about how her mom left her dad and left the kids with him and how he would always tell my wife she would never make anything of herself and that she was worthless. She said he was verbally abusive to her mom and that is why she left, and he took it out on her. I never thought highly of him after I heard that, but I dealt with it.

I did for Jordan as I did for my other two children growing up; they all got toys, and I took them to the movies as well. I found that when Jordan was a toddler, his mother wouldn't take him to the store, because he would grab things, so I ended up taking Jordan with me all the time. I gave him a nickname that has stuck until this day: he was dad's little Monkey Butt. I gave him this name because he was always hanging on me and going everywhere with me like Curious George.

As time progressed, things were not getting any better at work or at home, and I was told by someone it didn't matter how much education I had, a bachelor's or a master's degree—if they did not want to promote you, they could fudge the numbers on the interviews so your numbers would not be close enough. So, I figured since everything was political, I would take a different route in politics; I became a precinct committee man in my county, worked with our city and county, and assisted in elections for the state. I started putting up signs, assisting with dinners, and selling tickets and going to dinners to show my face and meet other politicians. I even assisted as county representative for the person that was running for governor. I felt good about this guy; he was attorney general for three terms, and he opposed our sitting governor for things he was doing. We needed a good person in the office.

So I became busy with work, taking care of the kids, and working on the governor's campaign in our county and a few surrounding counties as well. I slowly noticed a change in my wife: she wanted to go out with her friends more often, and she would not give me physical attention when I would try to hold her or cuddle her at night. Then, during that year, DCFS (Department of Children and Family Services) called to come over to the house and visit. I asked what it was all about, and they said there were allegations about my wife physically abusing my older kids. They came to my house to talk to me, and when they asked me about certain things, I could not give them an answer, because I was not home during the times they occurred. Well, the allegations were determined to be unfounded.

Jordan's Voice

Then one night, I got a phone call around midnight from a woman telling me that her husband and my wife were having an affair. The lady went on about their meetings and working late and private lunches. My wife asked, "Who is that on the phone?" I replied, "It's for you," and handed her the phone. She was screaming and yelling back and forth. Then my wife gave a stupid response out of anger to the lady: "If you were a better wife and you could satisfy him, this wouldn't be happening."

She hung up the phone, and I looked at her, saying, "So you are screwing your boss?" She replied, "No! I am not. She just made me angry, and I just had to say something stupid back to her." I got out of bed and went into the living room to sleep on the couch. I was angry, upset, and dumbfounded all at once. Somehow, I had a feeling something was going on, and I really didn't want to believe it, mainly because I didn't want to go through another divorce and split up my kids.

Several days went by. Then I went looking for this guy Steve, her boss. I had heard he was staying at an old motel in town. I went to the door, not knowing what I was going to say or do, so I knocked at the door, and when he opened it, he knew exactly who I was. I said to him, "Why?" and he replied, "I don't know; I don't love her." The next thing I did was tell him to stay away from my wife. Then I walked away. I mean, I could have punched him, but it was not worth losing my job over.

About a week went by, and he called me so I could hear what he and his wife had to say; they said they wanted to meet me and my wife at the police station in a public place so he could tell my wife it was all a game, and he didn't have feelings for her. My wife did not want me to go, but I did go, and she had her best friend go up there with her to the station. When we all arrived, we met out in the front lobby; Steve and his wife were with an officer there to keep everything civil. Steve, the guy who she was fooling around with, was the vice president of transportation at the company they worked for, and she would work late many times so they could fool around at the office. Steve did not waste any time and just came out and said to my wife, "It was all a game for me from the very beginning. I don't love you or have any feelings for you at all." My wife burst into tears with her best friend there to comfort her.

In a way, I was glad it hurt her. While she cried her heart out, I left and went back home, where my sister was watching the kids for me. When I arrived home, I thanked my sister for watching the kids, and she said, "Call me if you need to talk." I said OK back to her, she left, and I put the kids to bed. After I got the kids to sleep, I went into the bathroom and showered then headed to bed. It was not easy for me trying to sleep, and she had gone over to her best friends to spend the night.

I moved forward, trying to mend things at home. My candidate lost the election, and I just moved on. I was approached by one of the assistants of the candidate I was working for, asking me if I would run for county commissioner in my county. He said, "We need new and younger blood in this county" and thought I could do something. I sent off all my paperwork to make it legal. I wanted to do a respectable job for my county, plus if I won, then I would not have to work at the prison for a while. So I started getting contributions, making signs, and getting business cards made. I put a float together and placed it in the local parade, handing out balloons and candy to the kids. My kids and wife helped, and my father even drove his truck to pull the trailer. I really wanted this to work and to try to make a difference in my county and my family life—I wouldn't have such a long drive to work and could be home more.

Then after about a month, I started noticing a pattern at home: every night at the same time, she would go out on the deck to smoke and talk to someone. One night, I asked her, "Who are you talking to every night out on the deck?" She replied, "I'm talking to my best friend Barbra about work and what has been going on." Then one night, a couple of days later, when I was throwing something away in the trash, I saw her cell phone bill was all torn up in pieces, which was unusual for her and curious to me. Since she was not home (she was over at her best friend's house), I took the pieces out and put them together; I noticed that every night she called the same number at the same time and was on the phone for fifteen to thirty minutes.

So I called the number, and a woman answered, saying, "Dan's Landscaping and Lawn Service." I told her, "Ma'am, I must have dialed the wrong number," and hung up. I looked at all the numbers again, and

I dialed the number again slowly, to make sure it was right. A woman answered again, saying, "Dan's Landscaping and Lawn Service." I then asked, "Does a Steve work here?" and she said, "Yes. Do you need him?" I was furious and replied, "Yes. Can I talk to him?"

Steve picked up the phone, and I said, "What in the hell are you doing? You told her it was a game, and now you're back talking to her." He replied, "I did not contact her; she found out from a guy at work where I went after I was fired, and she tracked me down." I replied, "Then why talk to her if you don't care for her?" His final response was, "I don't know—it's a game to me." I then told him, "How can you live with yourself with five kids at home, one paralyzed from the waist down? And you have done this twice to your wife before."

I did not really understand his wife, but somehow, I did; it was all about the children and not breaking them apart. I hung up the phone and taped the phone bill together, then headed over to her friend's house, where she was hanging out with some other girls from the office. When I arrived, I went toward the backyard and approached her with the bill. She said, "What's this?" and I said, "It's over. You have been calling Steve for months." She began making excuses, so I left, and then I got on the phone to our county chairman and said I was stepping down from the race for county commissioner for personal reasons. I gave them back the money I had left, and any other items, they could use for another candidate. I felt if I could not keep my family together, I should not run for office.

So we separated for a while, and she stayed at the house of a friend from work, taking Jordan with her. He did not want to go and be away from his siblings; he was only three years old at this time. This lasted for about four months. The thing about all this was trying to keep it all together, going to work and being harassed, then coming home, trying to keep my kids in a better frame of mind as well. My older kids were glad she was gone; they were sad because their brother was not there, but they seemed to have a sense of relief from not dealing with her every day. I was getting tired of taking him back and forth from her friend's place to my house. He seemed happier with his brother and sister, and when I would drop him off, he would have a death grip around my neck, or she would have to pull him out of the vehicle to get him out. I would hear the same old thing: "You really taught him how to stage things. Bravo, good coaching with him." The thing was, I was not doing anything—that is how he felt.

So, the next time I picked him up, when it was time for me to drop him off, I told her, "I'm keeping him, and I'm filing for divorce tomorrow." She was upset and said, "You better not take him to the attorney's office." Well, I did not take him with me, but I left him with my dad and stepmother at their house then went straight to the attorney's office to explain the situation and get everything in motion. My attorney then said, "I will file this in the morning first thing." I left and headed back to pick up Jordan at my dad's house. When I arrived, I walked into the house and said, "Jordan." My stepmother seemed really upset and said, "Brad, he's not here; your wife came by about an hour after you dropped him off and said she wanted to see him." My dad then added, "She sat down, and he came in and sat on her lap. Then the next thing we knew, she had gotten up and said, 'There are no custody papers yet.' So she got up and left with him."

I did not know what to say or do at this point. My head was spinning. I called my attorney up and told him. He said, "Let me file the papers at the courthouse, and then we will go from there." The next day, I received a call from him: "I have good news and bad news. The good news is, I filed for the divorce; the bad news is, she had an attorney file a restraining order on you." I was like, "What?" He then said, "The court date for the restraining order is in two weeks, but there is no validity to her story, and there are too many holes in it." I was worried, because working in corrections, a restraining order could cause you to lose your job because you could not carry a weapon, but he reassured me it was going to get dropped, that it was a way for her to retain custody until the divorce was settled.

CHAPTER FIVE

The day of court for the restraining order came and went, just like my attorney had said, and now it was just a waiting game to get all the facts together and figure out the game plan. I went back into the house and was searching for the letter she wrote me about her father and anything else incriminating; there was a picture I found of her and her best friend out with a guy grabbing her boob. She would go out with her friends and come home around midnight or two in the morning, drunk and throwing up in the bathroom and at times passing out. The thing about all of this was, I missed being with my son, and so did his siblings. I was not eating much, and in a three-month period, I went from 238 pounds down to 180 pounds. I was talking about it with my fellow coworkers, and I could not focus very well on many things, then I had an hour drive home, and when I got home, I would cook dinner for my older kids and make sure they did their homework.

This went on, and I wanted to get it over with. My attorney did a deposition with my wife, and she agreed to everything, even coming home drunk, and my attorney grilled her about how she could have killed someone and caused a child to be fatherless or motherless. My attorney said I had a 90 percent chance of winning custody of my son. Then one day, I was called up to our warden's office; I thought it was for a temporary assignment as a counselor that I had put in for. I went straight to the office, and the secretary told me to have a seat. Then a guy from internal affairs stepped in and said to me, "What's up?" I then said, "I'm trying to get everything finished up with my divorce, and I have a great chance of getting custody of my son."

Bradley L. Lewis

The secretary told me to head back to the conference room. I walked back, and in the room were a male and female with badges on their waists. The male officer said, "Are you Bradley L. Lewis?" I said, "Yes, I am." The female officer said, "We are here because we were informed by a source that you were talking to an inmate's cellmate about a conspiracy of murder for hire." I looked at the officer and said, "What? I filed for divorce. I have done everything I am supposed to be doing, and my attorney says I have a ninety percent chance of getting custody of my son, so who has been blowing smoke up your ass?" The officer told me they already talked to the officer in my cell house, the inmate's wife, and my wife, and my wife said there was no way I would do anything like that. I was like, "No, I would not jeopardize the chance of getting custody of my son or lose custody of my other two children." Then they said they would get back to me if they needed anything else.

I left the office. I was in shock and didn't know what to think, but then later, I remembered a Level E (high escape risk) inmate said something to me one time, and it pissed me off. The inmate asked if I had "the package" because I had lost so much weight; in other words, he was asking if I had AIDS. I replied firmly, no. Then he began saying he had heard me talking to my fellow officers about what was going on with me. He went on, "You know there are people on the street that can take care of things for you?" I then looked at him and said, "That's my son's mom, and I wouldn't even consider something like that, so shut the fuck up." I left off the gallery pissed.

Then, a few days later, I was assigned to that gallery again, and the same inmate said, "Officer Lewis, man, I'm sorry for saying that. Can you accept my apology? I meant no harm, and I saw you were in a bad way." I said, "Forget it, and don't ask me about anything again." I was like, "That was that idiot that claimed that I blew that idiot off," but I should have written him up at the time. My mind was not focused on that; I just wanted to do my eight hours and go home. I told my mom, dad, and sister about it, as well as my attorney, so he would know before the divorce date got near.

Two weeks went by, and I was called up to internal affairs. The guy from internal affairs, who was in the room when the state officers were there interviewing me, said, "I got good news for you: the state officers finished their investigation, and they said it was unfounded." I was happy to hear that. He went on, "I need a final statement from you about what happened so that we can close our file."

I was thinking, "You were in there, and you heard everything that was said." I told him, "Let the guard hall sergeant come in during this, since he is our union vice president." He replied, "We're not investigating anything; we just need you to say what you told the state officers, and that's it." I then replied to him, "I would like the union vice president to come in here." He said again, "Officer Lewis, the state police are done, and we have to close up the allegation here."

I just wanted this over with so I could get my divorce, take care of my three kids, and try and live a normal life the best I could, so I told him the same things I told the state police and then left the office. The union vice president asked me how everything had gone. I said, "I kept asking for you, but he insisted that state police said it was unfounded and he needed me to say exactly what I told them." He did not like that he would not let him come in and said he should have written everything down at the time the state officers were there.

I left and went on my way back to the cell house; this was around the end of September, and I just continued forward, working, taking care of my kids, and waiting for the divorce to get over. At this point, it was hard for me to take care of all the bills at home, so I told the mortgage company I could not continue with the payments. I moved in with my sister after she called me and offered for us to move in with her. I had to begin figuring things out, so I talked with my wife and said, "We need to file for bankruptcy." We had a double mortgage because we had done repairs on the house, and she had four credit cards maxed out from her spending. The only thing we did not file bankruptcy on was our vehicles, which were needed to get to work, shop, and run the kids around.

Time went by, and in January, I was called to the assistant warden's office to sign some paperwork. When I arrived at the office, his secretary handed me a large yellow envelope that read "Employee Review Board."

I looked at the secretary and said, "What's this for?" She just said, "Sign for it, and you can see inside."

I walked out to the guard hall, and our union vice president asked me what was up. I showed him that they were sending me to the employee review board. We went to a side room and opened the yellow envelope and read the contents; they were charging me with socializing, conspiracy, and conduct unbecoming of an officer. The union president said, "This is ridiculous, and it seems they are finding a way to get rid of you." He went on, "Go back to your cell house, and we will figure this out."

I went home that evening and contacted a past associate director I knew. I took the packet to him to read. His reply to me after reading it was, "This is political from your time working on a governor's campaign and you running for precinct committeeman; you were on the wrong side of the aisle, and they want to make sure you have a black spot and can't do anything further." I was shocked and said, "Can they really do that?" And he replied, "Yes, and since I was associate director, I knew you were going to counseling and that you didn't approach the inmate, so this would have been a slap on the hand."

The thing about it was, it was not just a charge; it was my career, and I had already put eleven years into this rathole of a job. I told my mom, dad, and sister about it. I just couldn't believe what was happening. I looked back and realized that was why the guy in internal affairs did not want our union vice president to come in when he was talking to me. He lied and was told to manipulate me into regiving my statement. We went to the employee review board and made our statements. I said, "Even though captains and wardens sit in the barber shop talking to the inmates about personal things, you want to charge me with garbage when it was unfounded by a higher department of the state?" The meeting was over, and the union said they would appeal.

I left feeling less hopeful than before; it had become clearer they wanted me gone. No, I wasn't going to accept this. I knew I did not approach an inmate for any of the things that they were saying. I left, and the hour-long drive home did not allow any decompression for me. I was talking to God in my car and praying I would get through all this. When was my life going to get better than dealing with harassment from work, fighting in my divorce for custody of my son? This was a time in my life when I felt I was not really meant to be here on this earth, but in the back of my mind was, "I must think of my kids and take care of them."

Every day, I drove back to this place that wanted me gone and was still wondering when I was going to be walked out, because I did not know how hard the union was going to fight for me. I knew there was always a give-and-take with the union, and I had seen union presidents get promotions for agreeing with the administration on what they wanted to happen.

The day came. I was in one of the cell houses, and one of the officers said to me, "I heard someone up in the guard hall say they were going to walk you out after shift, that they were going to wait for the day shift leave." I received a call to head to the guard hall at 2:45 p.m. and wait until they called for me, so I waited and watched the shift leave, and I was called into the assistant warden of operations' office. I walked in, and he said, "Officer Lewis, please give me your badge and state ID. I'm notifying you that you're on a thirty-day suspension, pending discharge." I was pissed and I told the warden, "You haven't heard the last of me. I am going to fight this and sue this department."

The guard hall sergeant walked me out to the electric eye, and as I left, he said, "Good luck, Lewis." I got in my car and drove off. I was so mad, and I was crying. There were so many emotions going through me that I started praying to God to end this nightmare: "Lord, you know I'm not a mean or physical person and that I always fear trouble before even doing anything, so how could this be happening?" I really did not know what to do at this point or how I was going to tell my parents and explain to my kids why I would not be going to work anytime soon.

I waited a few days, then I decided to take charge of the situation and began calling the governor's office, explaining to them what happened and that state police said it was unfounded and the inmate lied. Then I said to them, "If nothing is done about this, I will go to *20/20* and let them know all about the parties at the warden's cottages with directors and deputy directors and female staff drinking and fooling around on state property."

I called every state senator and state representative about this. I left no stone unturned; I was not going to let them take my livelihood away all because everything was political across the state. My dad had me talk to our county chairperson, and I explained everything to him. He put me in the county highway department until I could get everything figured out, which helped a lot. I applied for unemployment, and I received a denial. When I called to appeal, they looked and said they were not paying it. I appealed it, and when the mediator called my house and had the representative from the state on the line, he asked the reason I was not being paid my benefits. The lady tried to give a spiel, but he asked if they had fired me, and she replied, "Yes." The mediator said, "You owe him his benefits—case closed."

I started working at the highway department right away so there were no interruptions with my bills, and I really needed assistance. I was going to a Baptist church before all this happened, trying to get things figured out, and there were people whom I had gone to school with in my Sunday school class. I thought when all this happened that people would call and pray for me, and only one replied; it was the pastor, who came over and prayed with me. I felt like, "Why are the people in my own Sunday school class judging me when everything was unfounded?" So, I quit going to church, but I wasn't giving up on God, and I had come to an understanding. When I filed for divorce, I went to one of the other vice presidents where she worked and told him of her affair and the shenanigans with her boss at work and the groundskeeper at the owner's house. I was taking vengeance, trying to get her fired, and God was showing me that I needed to be humble and let him do what he decided to do. It really hit me to the point that I cried for not being humble and not trusting in him to do the right thing.

Well, during this time, I tried keeping busy, and I met someone that I spent some time with. She told me what she did, and I told her what I did, but I left out the termination and what they tried to say I did. She was a nice person and wanted to be friends with benefits (FWB), which was a new concept to me. I mean, it seemed OK, but it was not really a clever idea for me, only because I began to get attached and have feelings for her. Then one day she said, "The three-bedroom duplex next to me is available; you could rent that, and we would be right next to each other." I had to explain to her what happened and that I was waiting for a third-level grievance, for an arbitrator to come in and make his decision. I explained that I had a past associate director, a state representative, and a state senator who were going to be at my hearing giving support and testimony on how it was an attack on me for being on the wrong side of the politics, which was the reason the situation had even gone this far. Then, as I thought she would, she said it was best we did not see each other, because she felt scared over the situation, not knowing everything. So we went our separate ways, and I did not look back.

I continued working with the county highway department. At the end of September, I received a call while at work on my cell phone; it was the union saying, "The state agrees to bring you back, but the thirty-day suspension stands, and they will pay you two months of back pay." I said, "Let me contact someone, and I will call you back." I called the past associate director and told him what they said. He replied, "Tell them ten days on the suspension and all your time back in pay." So I called the union back and told them, "Ten days suspension and all my back pay." I thought, "How much haggling are we going to do to come to an agreement?" The reply was, "Thirty days suspension and three months back pay." I told them I would call back, and I called the past associate director again and told him what they had said to me. The associate director understood the politics, because he was given the option to retire or be fired because he did not agree with the way they were running things. He replied, "Brad, I don't like it, because if you go back and they write you up and give you a one-day suspension, you're done; that's why they are strong-arming you. I know you want to get back to work for your kids as insurance for them." He continued, "The thing is, I just hope the arbitrator is out of state and hasn't been compromised."

I had a lot to think about. I called the union back and said, "I will agree, but are you going to go after them for unjust discharge?" They replied, "You have to get your own attorney to fight that." Then I said, "OK." I was told to return to work a few days later, and I thanked the county chairperson for the temporary work he had given me when I really needed it.

So I went back to work, and after two weeks, I received a letter in the mail from the Department of Corrections. I opened it up, and this is what it said: "The Department of Corrections agrees to reinstate Bradley L. Lewis as long as Bradley L. Lewis agrees he will not file any judicial actions against the state for unlawful discharge." It was signed off by the union. I was pissed and contacted the union and said, "What is this all about? You told me that you could not do anything about the unlawful discharge and that I had to get my own attorney." The union replied, "You wanted us to represent you, and we did." I then said, "You signed that, and I didn't; all you did was sell me out," and I hung up the phone.

So I returned to work as if I had never left, minus the money they owed me. I had to go six months walking on eggshells to not get written up for anything, but they also had to walk on eggshells to not harass me during this time. After about a month went by, a major said to me, "I knew you would be back; they were hoping you would not fight back, and you did."

I was mentally tired, and I went to my attorney and told him, "Let's get the divorce over with. I will agree to joint custody; my son stays with her." I couldn't drag it out. I was already in debt to him for $6,000, and I just wanted to take care of the kids the best I could; I stayed on the day shift so I could do this.

Time went by. The workdays came and went. They did their best to keep me from getting promoted, and to keep my mind off things, I would go out when I didn't have the kids and hook up with someone and just leave things at that. I did bring two people home with me—one I saw for three weeks, and the other I ended up being with for four and half years, and that was only because of her son—he was disabled, and I felt really sorry for him. Remember, I worked with special needs kids when I was a teacher's assistant after I got out of the military, and I felt I could do this. We were together for about a year, and she wanted to head up to Saint Louis, because that was where the children's hospital was; if something serious happened, he would be close. I agreed to move, and now my drive to work was an hour and a half. I began carpooling with fellow officers who lived up that way to save on gas. The bad thing was Jordan's mom moved from where they were an hour east. Now I would drive myself on Fridays an hour and a half to work, an hour and a half to pick Jordan up after work, and then an hour and a half to get home. Even if I didn't move, it would still be a four-hour drive.

I eventually put in for a transfer to a facility that was only a seventeen-minute drive from me under a hardship because of the other boy who lived with me. It was a new facility, but there were people there from the other facility, along with a major, and after a bit, I was hearing stories that I had tried to hire an inmate to murder my wife. I just wanted a fresh start, but people do not know how to leave things alone. Along with that, I did my best; there were a few times people tried to say I did things I did not do, but that was shot down.

I did jobs like road crew many times, and one day, while I had a crew out, the woman I was living with saw me on the road and pulled up and asked me for money for diapers for her son. I gave her the money and told her to leave before I got in trouble. Well, that did happen, and I told internal affairs that I did not tell her where I was, but her dad lived nearby, and when leaving his house, she spotted me and pulled over for money for diapers, and I gave her money and told her to leave. I started getting tired after a while of dealing with so many things with her and her older son. I just said, "Leave," but she did not until something happened and she had to leave.

By now, my older son had graduated, but I sent him back to his mom's. I sent my daughter, who had issues, back to her mom's as well. Kids think everything is greener on the other side until they find it is not. They were old enough to decide if they wanted to go back, and I was tired of the disrespect and not being appreciated for the things I did. I was in a house I bought with her and now had to figure out what to do, because the payments and bills were too much for me while paying child support for Jordan. So, I stopped paying the mortgage and put the house on a short sale; it took six months to sell, but I saved the mortgage money for a two-bedroom townhouse apartment for me and Jordan. I felt a lot better being by myself and decided to go back to school and take two classes;

they were on the same day, and I used upward mobility from work to pay for them. I was trying to finish my degree, but when I finished these two classes, I needed to take a math class—the problem being, math has always been my worst subject, and it is like learning Chinese for me. The degree dealt with behavioral psychology, another degree that allowed me to help people who had been born with disabilities or help those who had been injured get back to society and feel a part of the workforce. This was not the only reason for going to school; it was also to gain points in interviews to get promoted to sergeant. At every interview, there was a reason I was not promoted. One was they would never send me to inside training, and the sergeant on the tact team would not allow me to join either. These were must-have points, and they were holding training back. I started taking FEMA (Federal Emergency Management Agency) classes online and driving to places across the state for direct classes on my own time.

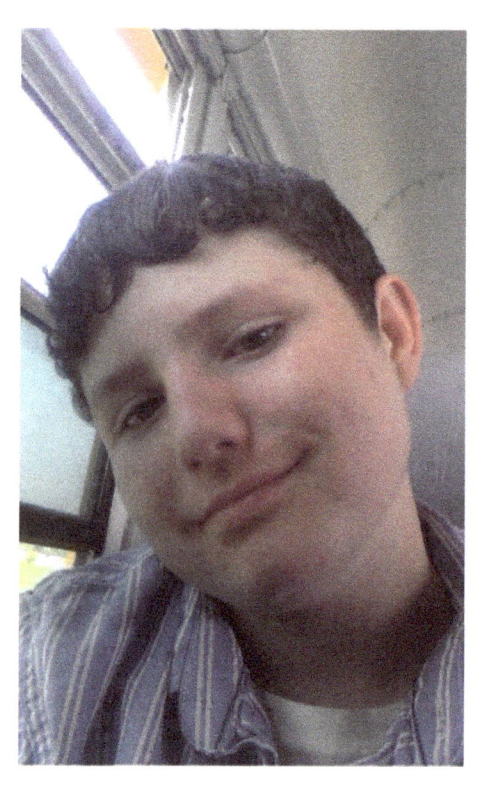

CHAPTER SIX

I was home on a Wednesday night. I gave Jordan a call—it was about 6:00 p.m.—and I told him that I found the *Fallout 3* game for him, along with the guidebook. I then told him, "Now you have me addicted to playing it." He replied, "It's not my fault," and I said, "I'm just joking with you. So I will see you Friday night."

The next morning, I went to work and was assigned the back door, where inmates signed out to work and go to horticulture classes. I got down there and had everything set up. I got a call at 7:30 a.m. from the armory, saying I had an outside call. They transferred the call to me, and I said, "Hello."

What I heard next sent shivers throughout my body. It was Jordan's mom; she was crying and said, "Jordan's dead."

I said, "What?"

She said, "Jordan's dead."

Then her best friend got online and said, "Brad, I'm really sorry, but Jordan shot himself, and he's dead."

She tried to explain, and I asked, "How did it happen?"

She replied, "He shot himself with my fiancé's shotgun, and the coroner along with the county sheriff have taken the body to the funeral home where they can prep him." But I couldn't focus, and I hung up.

I got on the radio and contacted my zone lieutenant to twenty-five my position ASAP, and I began screaming, "No, no, this isn't happening!" I started hitting the door and was still screaming.

The lieutenant and staff began running down the hall to where I was. They said, "What is wrong?"

I replied, crying, "My son is dead; he shot himself."

They quickly took my keys and radio, and two of the staff were told to drive me home. When I got home, I called the woman I was dating and told her about what happened; she left work and headed to my house. I had already changed clothes, and when she arrived, we headed down to the county he lived in. While driving, I called the county sheriff's office and was transferred to the lead detective on my son's shooting. I asked for all the details, and he replied, "He left a suicide note." He couldn't remember what it said, but he knew it mentioned that he was bullied and that was the reason why he did it.

I had so many emotions going through me that I was struggling to sort them out, hoping I could maintain and control them so the wrong ones would escape and cause more pain and suffering to anyone having anything to do with his death. My focus was getting there and seeing his body and then figuring out the funeral arrangements. I called my stepmother and told her, and she was upset. I asked her, "Can I have the plot next to my dad so he can be buried there?" and she agreed. I did not have any plots paid for, and I knew my son had been with me to visit my father's grave many times; he was a pallbearer at my father's funeral, filling in for me. My father passed away on December 5, 2011, and Jordan saw all the pain and suffering my father experienced before he died.

I called my mom on the way down while my girlfriend was driving. When I told her Jordan was dead, I felt my mom's heart crumble as she cried out, "What, Bradley? Jordan is dead?" All I heard was tears and cries of pain. Along with all those memories of losing her son little Roger Jr. to drowning, it made her stomach drop and her heart heavy with grief hearing that my baby boy had died. She started asking how it happened as she cried. I didn't know how to tell her as the tears filled my eyes and my lips gripped tight together. Then it came out: "Mom, he shot himself with a shotgun."

She began asking questions that I had no answers to yet. I then said, "Mom, I have to let you go for now, because I have to call work for the life insurance and then call and see if I can find out anything." I made it down to my sister's house, and as I headed into the garage, there was my mom, a frail older woman in her mid-seventies, standing there with her eyes red and tears running down her face. She hugged me, saying over and over, "I wish with all my heart that Mama could bring back your baby. I know how you're feeling, son."

My heart ached, and it felt like someone had reached in and stolen part of my soul. I did not cry; even though my eyes were filled with tears, I was holding back. My girlfriend and I went in, along with my mom. Then my niece and her husband came by with my brother and my daughter and her boyfriend. I called the state attorney's office and the lead detective on my son's case to find more answers. Then I called the funeral home to set up a time to go with his mother to make arrangements and view his body. The main thing going through my mind was, "Where did he shoot himself, and did he suffer?" The other big question I was pondering was whether God would accept him into heaven. He was a child, and he did what he did out of pain and fear, I assumed, since the suicide note said he was bullied. I had always believed that if you took your life before God decided it was your time, you would go to hell. I knew God was a forgiving God, but could he allow us to enter heaven when we were being weak and doing something at the same time we were asking for forgiveness?

When my brother sat down after arriving, he told me a friend of his daughter had gone to school with Jordan, and she had given him names of kids who she knew were bullying him. My brother said, "She mentioned the name of one boy who told him the day before, 'Jordan, you don't have the balls to go home and kill yourself.'" She also said that the boy did not return to school the next day. I was angry. My heart was beating so hard, I felt like ripping someone apart, but then another side of me wanted to find out every detail of what, where, when, why, and how!

There was not time to cry now, but I was thinking about what I needed to do, so while everyone sat crying, all I wanted to know was who had pushed him to do this. Then my girlfriend and I headed out to the funeral home, and there, I met Jordan's mom. She had her sister, aunt, and niece with her. His mom and I sat and talked to the funeral director, who went over the basics and asked where he was going to be buried. I said, "Next to his grandfather and my older brother." Even though she wanted him in her family plot, I insisted that he would want to be by his grandpa.

We then went in to pick the vault and casket we wanted so they could finish cleaning his body for us to view. Jordan's favorite color was blue, so it was not hard to pick a color, but I wanted a Christian theme with crosses on all four corners and a spiritual quote on the top inside lining. Jordan's mom really did not want a church atmosphere, and she stated that to the director. I knew she never let Jordan go to church even though he wanted to go with Grandpa and Grandma, so, I guess, why would she change now?

From there we finished and headed over to the next room, where he was ready for us to see him. They had a white T-shirt on him and a sheet covering his bottom half. They had placed a hard shell over his heart where he shot himself, with the same on his back. I was in tears and trying to be nice. I patted his mom's back to give comfort. It was hard to see him like this, knowing he and I had plans that weekend and at the end of October to watch the Chicago Bears in Saint Louis. Then I started wondering again, "Did he suffer, or was it a quick death?" I know he was suffering inside, because why would you do this if you were not hurting? And what, or who, pushed him to this level of insanity, doing something like this?

Jordan's mom leaned over and gave him a kiss and stood back up. I looked down and placed my hand on his, feeling the coldness from him. He looked so peaceful, as if he were asleep lying there, but his body was asleep, and now in front of us was an empty vessel of who he had been. I placed my hand on his mom's back, and as she turned, I gave her a hug and said, "Why? Why did he do this?" She replied, "I don't know why." I then turned and gave him a kiss on his head and said, "I love you, Monkey Butt. You did not die in vain, and I will find out who did this and make sure it does not happen again."

We were in there for about twenty minutes. Then we turned and walked out. We were not going to allow anyone else to see him like that, and I needed to head out and pick an outfit for him. They said a shirt, tie, and a suit jacket were all we needed. I cried, but not the way I wanted to. You could tell I was holding a lot back. My girlfriend and I headed back home so I could plan with work for time off and get things together for the funeral. I continued to call people, but that night after my girlfriend left, I went to my room, took my meds, and turned on the television until I fell asleep.

The next morning, I called work, then called the state attorney's office, the Board of Education for the state, and the lady who deals with state insurance and got the paperwork rolling. I then heard that on Wednesday, the day before Jordan took his life, the school had shown an antibullying movie toward the end of the day, in the last hour, in the gymnasium. I did remember when driving back home that I called my son's high school to talk to the principal, and when he answered, I told him, "The first thing you need to do is find out what kids bullied Jordan." Then I asked, "Did you view the movie that was shown to the kids? Has the superintendent even seen it?" The principal said, "No! I did not see the movie, and I was not at the school when they showed it." I replied, "You better not show that movie again, unless it is something approved by the Board of Education and parents give their permission for their kids to view it." I then told the principal that if he did not do his job, I would have the media focused on his school, wondering what happened at the school he oversaw.

I started gathering pictures so they could put a video together, showing Jordan coming into this world and the last photo of him taken before taking his life. While looking through the pictures, I saw all the ticket stubs for concerts, football games, and baseball games we attended; my mind was about ready to explode with all the good memories I had with my son. That is when I decided to go online and make a video to say what I wanted to say, so I could clear my head a little. The video was nothing planned, but pure emotions came out of me, pouring like running water. When I finished, I did not bother viewing it; I just loaded it up to my YouTube account and Facebook and shared it with everyone. I wanted to share how I was feeling and hoped I could get some answers so this would never happen again to anyone else's child.

I sat back in my recliner, and what I began thinking was far from what I should have been thinking: it was what my mom feared I might ponder and what my girlfriend knew in some ways might be going through my mind. The thoughts boggled my mind, and I began to cry, "How could he do it? How had he made sure he was so precise that he would kill himself immediately to not suffer?" I tried picturing in my mind how he did it. Did he pull the trigger himself? Tie a string to the trigger? Or did he aim it exactly right and use something long to push the trigger while he held the shotgun? I must have sat in that chair for hours, thinking of that vision in my head. I was very tired, and I showered, filled my CPAP, took my meds, and laid down in bed. I prayed to God with tears filling my eyes for him to give me strength, patience, wisdom, knowledge, the voice to speak, perseverance, and anything else I needed to allow me to take a stand and be Jordan's voice and the voice of other children who have suffered and still are suffering. Then I laid there, holding my son's stuffed monkey which I had bought him, feeling like I was holding him for the last time, and I held it tight until I fell asleep.

The next morning around 9:00 a.m., I dragged myself out of bed, went to the bathroom, and headed downstairs to get something to eat and drink. My head was cloudy; I still did not want to accept my little buddy was gone. But once I got my head together, I headed back up to my desk in my bedroom and began making phone calls again. I was calling everyone I could think of who I could get involved with this situation. I was not going to accept that my son had done this unless he felt there was no hope, and I could not rest until the truth was out there. I called the attorney general's office, local state senators, and our local state representative; I called the Board of Education, and they said, "We are going to call the state police headquarters down by where your son lived and have them do an investigation."

I then called a state representative for my district, asking what his views were on bullying in the state school system. He replied, "I'm against any school harassment or violence, and I will look into what the state bill says about it." Then I logged onto my computer, to Facebook. I noticed I was getting several replies from people from different areas of the county my son had resided in telling me how sorry they were to hear what had happened. I was getting messages from kids telling me the names of the kids that were bullying my son and telling me that one kid on the football team last year walked up behind him in the locker room and punched the back of his head from behind for no reason except that he was mad.

Jordan's Voice

The kid continued, "Jordan reacted, and when the coach came in, he gave Jordan detention and made the other kid run laps so he could still play in that week's football game and Jordan could not." Then a parent said Jordan told them he went to the principal's office about it, and all the principal did was side with the coach and tell Jordan to grow up and quit being such a crybaby. The parent did not want me to use their name, because they were afraid of the repercussions from the school system on their children and the politics in the community. The person gave me their number, and I called them and talked to them; they knew Jordan, as he had come over to their house several times to play with their child. They said, "Start at the top, because the principal does a lot of covering up and bullying of kids himself." I thanked the parent for the info and began viewing more messages from kids, then I came across others talking about Jordan being bullied.

One child said she heard a boy tell Jordan the day before that he didn't have the balls to go home and kill himself. I remembered my brother told me a friend of his daughter had said that and had not come back to school the next day. I could not believe what I was hearing: a principal bullying kids and covering up bullying, a football coach hiding behavior issues on his team and taking care of the better players, then a kid telling my son he does not have the balls to go home and kill himself. How much more was I going to hear? And still, I had to begin sending pictures of Jordan to the funeral home, give them the names of the pallbearers on my side of the family, and let them know the music I wanted played.

I called Jordan's mom as well to tell her about the video I posted and the responses from other children and parents about Jordan being bullied, but the response I received was not what I expected. Or was it? She was angry and would not listen to a word I said. All she said was, "Take the video down. The school is upset about it, and it is going to make Jordan look bad."

I replied, "If we don't find out who bullied him and put a stop to it, then it will just continue!" His mom was screaming at me, in tears, "Just take it down! It will make Jordan look bad!" Then her brother got on and said, "Brad, take that video down now." I just hung up. I was not going to listen to someone telling me to stop looking or to not find out what happened to my son! I quit calling people and began getting my clothes together then had to run to the store to find a tie, pants, dress shirt, and shoes to wear at the funeral. I ran around to several places and found what I needed. I hadn't dressed up since my dad's funeral, and I didn't want a suit jacket, because I had no time to get one fitted. Jordan wore the homecoming outfit I bought him: a white shirt, a blue tie with the Chicago Bears emblem as a tie clasp, and black pants. I did not have to buy a tie; I wore the Chicago Bears tie Jordan bought for me for Father's Day.

I was losing track of time, so I rushed home to wash my clothes and pack for the weekend. My girlfriend and I were going to head out around 7:30 a.m. Saturday and stay the night in a hotel, then go to the wake and funeral on Sunday and head back home afterward. My girlfriend arrived at my place after work, around 5:30 p.m. We made sure we had everything we needed and packed it into the vehicle so there would be no rushing the next morning. She helped me a lot to remember things I might have missed. In addition to God collaborating with me, keeping me together, she gave me a lot of support when needed.

That evening, Mom called me to see how I was doing, in tears, her voice quivering with each word she spoke. "Are you all right, son? Mom worries about you. I didn't sleep a wink last night, and your brother has names from a friend's daughter who went to school with Jordan." I already knew about the girl who had given my brother the names, but my heart ached for my mom, knowing it was tearing her up inside seeing me lose my son at a youthful age as she had lost her son. I told my mom I would be down there in the morning after I stopped by my stepmom's house. I got off the phone and checked the computer; more people had sent comments about the bullying and how they had been bullied as well. The entire day wore me out, so I went into the bathroom and shaved and took a nice, hot shower to try and relax. When I finished, I put on my nightclothes and laid down to fall asleep.

The morning came quickly. We were up and dressed, and we headed out. I decided to drive since I had no one else to call that early in the morning. The drive was quiet at first, and my girlfriend turned on some music since I was not much into talking; I was sorting things out in my mind.

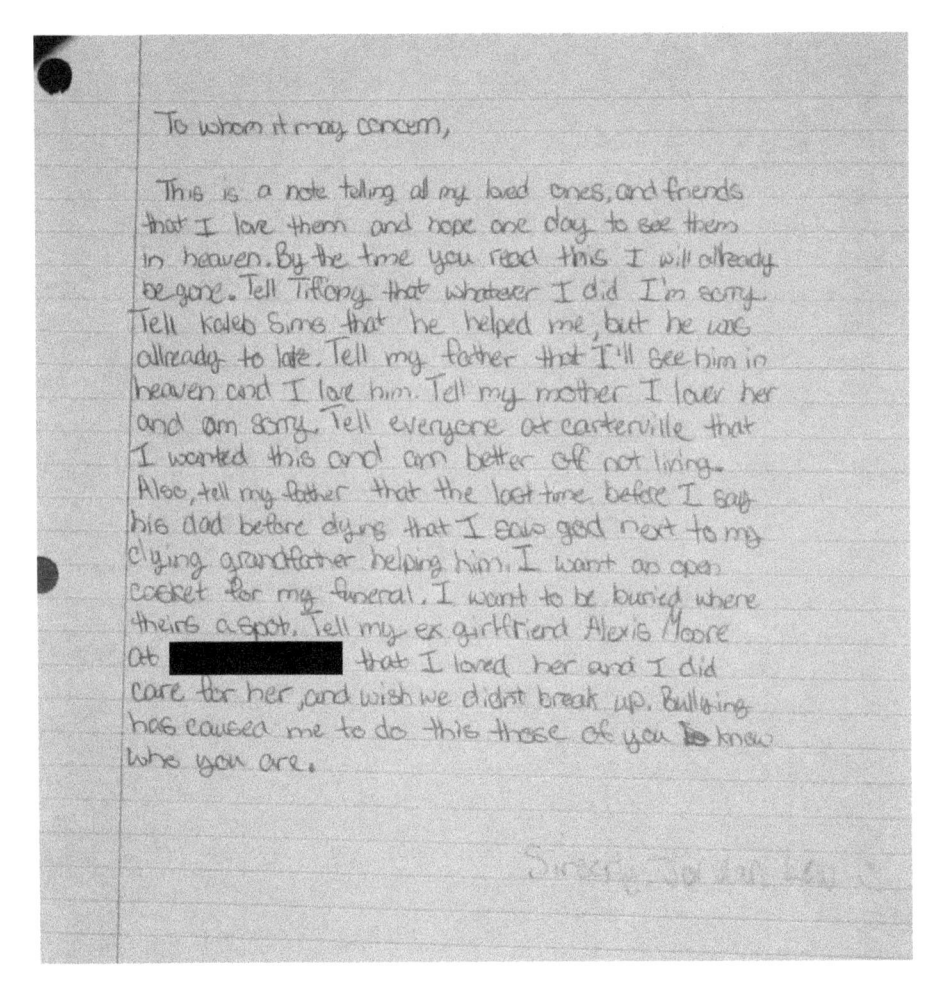

> To whom it may concern,
>
> This is a note telling all my loved ones, and friends that I love them and hope one day to see them in heaven. By the time you read this I will already be gone. Tell Tiffany that whatever I did I'm sorry. Tell Kaleb Sims that he helped me, but he was already to late. Tell my father that I'll see him in heaven and I love him. Tell my mother I love her and am sorry. Tell everyone at carterville that I wanted this and am better off not living. Also, tell my father that the last time before I saw his dad before dying that I saw god next to my dying grandfather helping him. I want an open casket for my funeral. I want to be buried where theirs a spot. Tell my ex girlfriend Alexis Moore at ████████ that I loved her and I did care for her, and wish we didn't break up. Bullying has caused me to do this those of you know who you are.
>
> Sincerely, Jordan ███

This was the suicide note Jordan left so people would understand why he did this and so he could say goodbye to those he loved.

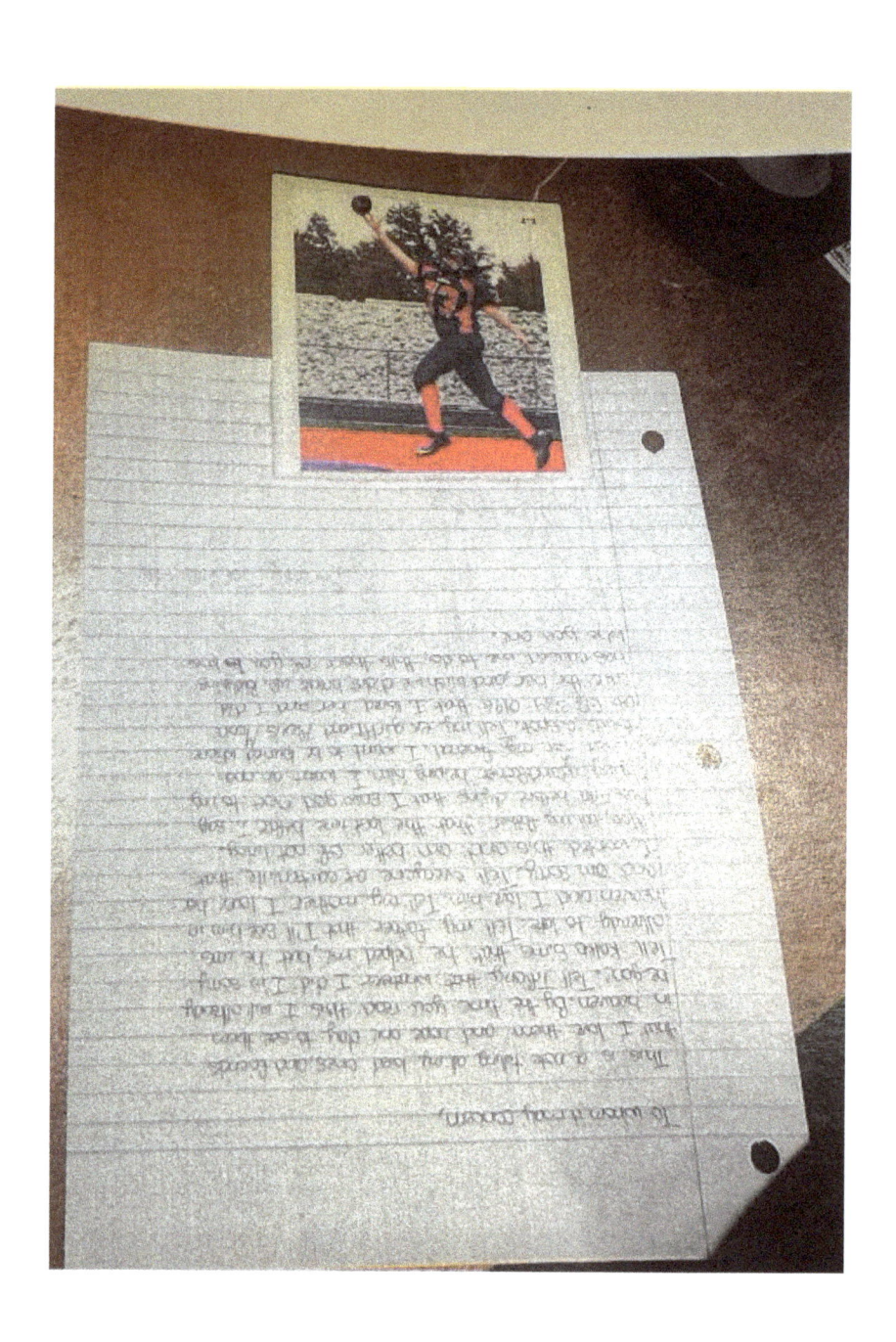

CHAPTER SEVEN

What was on my mind? Many things, but mostly the good times Jordan and I had going places and doing things. Then I started thinking about the games I purchased tickets for and concerts that he would never be able to go with me to see. I had tears building up, but I just kept a strong face and kept driving. My girlfriend would still look over occasionally and ask, "Are you OK?" I would look over and say, "Yes."

I knew I had several things to do, because Channel 3 had called and wanted to do an interview with me about Jordan's death and a video I had posted on YouTube and Facebook. I arrived in town and first stopped at my stepmom's house. We visited for about forty minutes and then headed to my sister's house, where the family was. I was shocked; this was the first time we had all been together at my sister's house, and it was sad that it took the death of an innocent little boy to bring the family together. There were no fights between us; I loved my family, but it was just that there was a large generation gap, and everyone had their own interests and beliefs. I thought it was nice to see us all together like this, but Jordan and the fact that this had happened to him were on my mind a lot. My brother tried talking to me, giving me the names on a piece of paper of the boys who were bullying Jordan, which had been given to him by a friend's daughter, who went to school with Jordan.

I received a call from a young girl Jordan went to school with at his old school, and she said, "Mr. Lewis, me and Jordan were like boyfriend and girlfriend when he went to school there; we did not go out, but we talked on the phone a lot." She added, "I talked to Jordan the night before he committed suicide, and he was breaking it off with me and said he needed to deal with his issues and that he loved me. I was scared. After he hung up, I told my grandmother about it, and we did not know a number to reach you or his mother, so my grandmother called the police station where he lived and told them Jordan's name and his address and what he was going to do. Supposedly the cops went by and did a wellness check."

I thanked her and told her I would get back to her soon. After I got off, I told my family what this girl had said, and my family said, "Why did they not do anything? And if his mom knew they were there talking to her, why did she go to work the next morning, leaving him alone?" There were so many questions from everyone, and I knew there were going to be many more, some I could answer and some I had no answers to, but I was determined to find out all I could from whoever I could get the information from.

At this point, my girlfriend and I had to head out; I had appointments with Channel 3 and Channel 12. I knew I had time for one interview, and the other had to wait till later. I then headed over to my daughter Deeanna's place and asked if they had anything decent to wear. She said no, so I drove them to the store and bought them something appropriate for a funeral. We dropped my daughter off back at her house, then headed back to my sister's house and sat down to eat. When we were finished, we all went to the family room and sat watching a movie and talking to one another.

It was getting late, so my girlfriend and I headed back to the hotel she had booked for us. We showered and laid out our clothes for the funeral and burial and went to bed. Sunday morning came early, it seemed. I woke up saying, "Good morning, God, Jesus, my dad, and now Jordan." Then we began getting dressed and packing everything up and checked out of the hotel. Before going to the funeral home, we stopped off at Kroger so I could pick up three dozen red roses for the cemetery, so each family member could put a rose on the casket as they walked by to say their last goodbye.

We arrived at the funeral home and parked where they asked us to, then headed in with a couple of trays of meat, cheese, and plates we had bought. We sat the food in the sitting area out of the way, then I went into the funeral home's office to make sure to print a few extra memorial videos to give my mom, daughter, and sister. I walked back into the room where Jordan was laid out, then I took a Chicago Bears scarf and draped it off the side of the casket and placed his favorite stuffed monkey at the base of the casket. So much was going on that I forgot that Jordan's mom had arrived right after we did, and when I tried talking to her about finding out who bullied our son, she just jumped right back at me, saying, "It doesn't matter now; it won't bring him back. Do you want those kids locked up, ruining their lives, for a mistake?" I said, "I don't want this to happen to any other child or have a parent suffer a loss that could be prevented." She just walked away, and I never had any backing from her or her family in getting information about who bullied Jordan.

I went back in and stood by Jordan's casket, viewing him with my mother, sister, and daughter. My son arrived, and he came into the viewing area, stopping about ten feet away from the casket, and stood there for about five minutes, then he turned and left. I had asked him to be a pallbearer, but he said no. I really did not understand—unless it was all the times, I asked him to go to concerts and ballgames with me and Jordan but he was too busy. I stayed up front by the casket, greeting people as they came in and paid their respects, but I was an empty shell. I do not know how I was making it, but God was giving me the strength to stand and greet everyone, thanking each one for coming.

During the time I was greeting, a lady walked up to me and said, "Mr. Lewis, I just want to tell you the police dropped the ball; they should have contacted child services or even taken him to an emergency room to have an evaluation done for a wellness check so they would be OK to be left alone." I told the lady thank you and continued greeting. Then a large group of kids from Jordan's school began walking in. I began greeting each of them separately, away from Jordan's mom, and thanking them for coming. One girl came up to me and said, "That one boy turned himself in and is in juvenile detention," but I didn't know if that was true; there would be so many stories I would have to sift through, as if they were grains of wheat, to see which ones were valid. More people started coming in, then the pastor who was going to do the service came in as well, then the young lady who Jordan went to homecoming with asked if she could say a few words, but Jordan's mom would not allow it. Jordan's mom said, "The kids can have their own time at their own get-together." Nothing had changed with Jordan's mom—still the same old center-of-attention person; whether it was positive or negative, she wanted the attention.

More people poured in to pay their respects. If only Jordan could have seen those three to four times as many people attended his funeral as had attended his grandpa's. I wish he could have seen how many people missed him and loved him compared to the few who bullied him. I noticed a friend of mine, Elizabeth, had come all the way from the West Saint Louis area, from around Ballwin, to pay her respects; she never met Jordan, but she felt like she had, given how much I would talk about him. There were several of Jordan's mom's family members and friends there, but I never saw his mom's fiancé standing by her giving her any moral support during the funeral. I did put my hand on her back and pat her to give her some moral support, even though there were mixed emotions about what she thought about me posting the video online. Then I noticed in the mix of people coming through was my warden; he had made the two-hour drive to give his respects as a representative for my institution. I shook his hand and said, "Thank you, Warden, for coming; it means a lot receiving your support." I was not happy to see him and wished they had sent someone else, but he was the warden, and he made that call. I had had issues with management ever since my last institution, where they terminated me unlawfully and kept me from suing them, but this warden never wanted to promote me because I would not kiss his butt like others did.

After the rest of the people came through, they had to set up chairs in the outer area with all the partitions opened. The pastor stepped up and asked everyone to be seated so he could start the service, thanking everyone for being there, and then introduced Jordan's aunt on his mother's side to read a poem she had written. The poem was nice and spoke of forgiveness and how we should not carry a weight of anger because Jordan was in a better place. She went on, but I cannot remember everything she said. I barely watched the video with all the pictures showing Jordan from when he was a baby up until he was in sports; his mom sent me a couple of pictures of him at baseball, but that was all I received. I received newspaper clippings from a lady from the other town they lived in, and that was more than what I received from Jordan's mom. I mean, I offered to pay

Jordan's Voice

but never received anything. That was just like when I picked him up on my weekends—she would never make an effort to drive him back, except one time when I had to have surgery on my knee. She had to drive him to me, and she said, "This is the last time I do this," even though she was supposed to share in the driving. I even had problems with her sending clothes on the weekends. She'd only send the set he was wearing, and that was it. I would have to buy him clothes for my house, and I would wash the pair she sent and let him wear them back. I knew Jordan wanted to take some back because they were name brands, so I would let him when he was in junior high; it made him happy that he picked out his own, and it made him feel like he fit in with other kids. Jordan wanted to look nice, and he really wanted to fit in with the cool kids. He was a special person who wanted to be friends with everyone and be liked by everyone. I was told by a kid in his class that Jordan was a person who would try and make you laugh and always ask you how you were doing, and if you were feeling bad, he would try and cheer you up. Another kid mentioned to me, "I never saw him mistreat anyone, because he wouldn't want no one to mistreat him."

So, during the service, I just looked at him while sitting next to my daughter, thinking about the things he wanted to do after he graduated high school. One was going into the service and earning his college money so he could go to college like I did. The pastor stepped up and performed a short but heartfelt service, asking the younger group to look toward God. When he concluded, they ushered people through so they could say their last goodbye seeing his sweet, peaceful body lying there before permanently closing the casket and letting go of his earthly shell. When everyone had left, they sealed the casket and rolled it to the front door, where my brother, my niece's husband, Jordan's mom's brother, a good friend of Jordan's, Jordan's mom's dad, and I lifted the casket and placed it in the hearse. We all went to our vehicles to follow the hearse to Jordan's final resting spot, next to his grandpa and his uncle. When we arrived, I took out the three dozen roses and gave one to each of the immediate family members that were there. The pastor said a final prayer, and then each person with a rose placed it on his casket and said goodbye.

Some family members took flowers that were in his casket when they closed and sealed it so they could go home and press them in a book. I said my final prayer, then said, "Goodbye, little Monkey Butt," and I swore I would spread his voice abroad. My girlfriend and I said goodbye to the family, then we headed back out to the Saint Louis area. During our drive back, I was going through my Facebook messages and noticed there were more responses to my video, which had gone viral. There were many messages of people giving their condolences and letting us know they were praying for our family because of our loss. I then came across a person who wanted to contact me by phone and said they were told by the Holy Spirit to lend a hand and help us make people more aware of the problem of bullying. I told my girlfriend what the person had said, and she replied, "That is nice, but you have to be careful, because a lot of times, people will feed off people who are grieving and take advantage of them." I said, "I know. I will call the person tomorrow and find out more about what they want to do." I then told my girlfriend that the money was collected in the drop box and that she should keep all the money she received from her friends and family and not give it to me to help pay for the headstone.

When we finally arrived back at my place, I helped my girlfriend place her suitcase into her vehicle and gave her a hug and kiss good night. I watched her pull away, then I shut my garage door, made my way to the laundry room, and threw a load of clothes into the washer. I headed upstairs to the kitchen to grab something to drink and then to my bedroom. I placed the envelopes the funeral home had given me on my desk along with the memorial video and proceeded to take a shower and put my sleeping clothes on. After that, I sat back in my recliner and relaxed until I went to bed. I had taken medicine to help me sleep, but it was not working. As I held Jordan's stuffed monkey, my eyes filled with tears. I tried praying, and even though I did not have to speak but rather say the prayer in my head, even the words in my head were boggled up. I cried to God, asking him to give me the strength to fight back at Satan for what he did by taking my son away. The memories of my little buddy ran through my mind, of him lying in the casket and of me touching his hand for the last time. I eventually fell asleep and was out for the night; this was the

Jordan's Voice

most emotional strain I have ever had in my life, given how much energy it took out of me.

Monday morning came. I dragged myself out of bed, going to the bathroom and washing my face to wake myself up. I went to my computer to view new text messages people may have sent me, to see if there was any additional information. I read several texts and was amazed by the names of kids and what had transpired in the past year. Besides my son being bullied, parents were telling me of their own altercations and how the school would do nothing about it. This was from my son's school, but there were others from surrounding counties as well as kids having trouble. Then I came across a text from a woman who lived in my son's town; she gave me the number of a lady looking to get ahold of Jordan's dad. I called the number she gave me, and the phone rang. Then a woman picked up and said, "Hello." I said, "Hi. I'm Brad Lewis, Jordan's father." She said, "I'm Jacqueline Rose, and I'm from a CNN morning show." She began saying how sorry she was for what happened and my loss, and then she said, "We would like for you to fly out this evening and be able to do the morning show with Chris Cuomo; we will fly you out and put you up in a hotel across from the studio and fly you home the next day." I told the lady that I had never been to New York, and I had not flown in a plane in twenty years, so I had to ask if I could bring someone since I was still coping with my son's death. The lady said, "That would be fine; we understand." I called my girlfriend, and she agreed about me traveling alone and not knowing how to get around, so she put in for the next day off from work, then left work early and headed to her house to pack.

I started getting my clothes together and figuring out what I needed to take. Between all the preparation, I was still making calls trying to get more information, even calling the federal Department of Education in Washington. I explained the situation to someone in this department. They took my info and were going to give it to another person who would contact me back. Then I noticed online the interview from Saturday before the funeral; I could not believe how quickly everything was happening. I know just a week before we had been talking about a young girl in Florida who took her life due to being bullied—she jumped from the top of a grain silo, falling from an extremely elevated position onto concrete.

I knew Jordan wanted to live with me because he would say it all the time, and I knew he begged his mom to let him live with me. He got tired of asking, but I wondered if that was why he was being so persistent this year—all the bullying and wanting to get away from it. I just wished I could get all the answers and piece it together so that something like this did not happen again and changes could be made. I called the lead detective on my son's case, telling him I had received information from kids and parents on Facebook, but I wasn't able to get through to him. Then I tried contacting the county state attorney's office and stated my complaint and asked if they would check in on it. The lady in the office said, "I will pass the info on to one of the state attorneys."

Time was slipping away with all the calling. It was almost 3:00 p.m., and I still had to pack my CPAP machine and get my meds and computer packed up along with the memorial video and pictures of Jordan. I called Jacqueline Rose back and confirmed the information, then texted my girlfriend the flight information along with Jacqueline's number so she could make sure we were confirmed on the flight that night. It was going to be a rush getting to the airport, finding a parking spot, then catching a shuttle bus and checking our baggage in before the flight. I would have been so lost, but since my girlfriend had traveled so much with her job and knew all the ins and outs of traveling, things went a lot better. The flight was going to be two hours long, and with New York being an hour ahead of us, we would lose an hour. The flight headed out at 9:05 p.m. and would arrive just after 10:00 p.m. their time, so by the time we got our baggage and drove to the hotel, it would be around 11:30 p.m.

My girlfriend made it home, packed her stuff, and called her mom, so if her phone died, her mom could call my phone, then left and headed to my place, where we packed our things in my vehicle and headed to the airport. I wanted to leave a little early so we would have no traffic or hiccups along the way. We grabbed something to eat at the airport and used the restroom before the boarding call. I was nervous—one, because I was going on national television to tell my son's story of bullying, and two, I had not flown in twenty years.

I would state only what I knew or repeat what kids or parents had told me; I was not going to state my opinion. Then there was the important thing of giving only titles and not names of people. The reason is, you cannot give names of minors out, and you cannot give the names of people who may be involved—only attorneys or police can. I wanted to make sure Jordan's voice would be heard in a positive format. Then people would take bullying more seriously rather than thinking it was just a part of life.

The call came through the speaker to board the plane. We grabbed our carry-on baggage and went down the walkway onto the plane. I was shocked, as I thought it would be bigger inside. I mean, yeah, after twenty years they still had people crammed together like sardines. I sat by the window and prepared myself for takeoff. I reached up to turn on the air, and it did not come on. My girlfriend said, "It doesn't come on until the plane starts moving." Then she asked, "Are you all right?" I replied, "Yes." It seemed some things about flying had not changed for me—I still needed the air blowing in my face. I wiped down my window and placed my face against it while taking off; since they do not clean these planes down very well before ushering people off and back in them, you do not know who coughed or sneezed on that window.

Before I knew it, we were in the air, and I was looking down at all the lights of all the houses and highways surrounding Saint Louis. As we circled, we climbed higher in altitude, and then we were above the clouds. My girlfriend was in a conversation with a younger gentleman next to her. I didn't mind—I wasn't much of a conversationalist at the moment. I placed my earbuds in my ears and started listening to songs on my playlist. I was doing well until I came across Bon Jovi and "Army of One" began to play. I started tearing up a little, because Jordan and I had gone to a Bon Jovi concert at Scottrade Center in Saint Louis that year. I do not believe he sat down the whole concert; some older guys behind us gave him a high five and said, "He's got good taste in music." I smiled at him, and when the concert was over, we headed to our vehicle and back to my place. Jordan leaned over in the vehicle and said, "Dad, I love you." That made me feel good inside—the cost of the floor seats was worth that appreciation. That was not the only concert we had gone to that year. We also saw Ted Nugent, Styx, REO Speedwagon, and Mötley Crüe, then later in the summer, we saw Kenny Chesney at Live Nation out in Earth City, Missouri. We had a blast that summer. Along with going to three baseball games—the Cardinals versus the Cubs—we went on long bicycle rides, about seventy-three miles, and we still had one main item scheduled in late November, and that was the Chicago Bears versus the Rams; that was never going to happen.

During the flight, I was pretty zoned out with the music and the memories and how much I was missing him not being there and not being able to watch him fulfill his dreams. I would pop in and out of my thoughts, and my girlfriend was still in full conversation with the guy next to her. I had to get up and use the restroom—or try. Wow! When I opened that door up, there was hardly any room to get in or turn around. I felt sorry for those who attempted to join the Mile High Club in that thing. I accomplished the task with precise movements so there were no incidents and cleaned my hands in the tiny birdbath sink, then went back and sat down. I talked to my girlfriend a bit and ordered a soda. Just like the bathroom, the can was so small; I took two drinks, and it was gone. I then laid my head back for a bit until I heard over the intercom, "Turn off all electrical devices and place your seatbelt on. We are on approach to New York." I turned my iPod off and looked out the window at all the lights around the city as we began our descent. As the plane was getting closer to landing, I grabbed my seat, anticipating the wheels touching the ground. Contact was made and the jets placed in reverse to slow the plane.

We made it to the terminal, and as we exited the plane, I followed my girlfriend, who knew her way around New York and the airport, to the baggage area. As we headed that way, we ran into Jacqueline Rose, who was waiting for us. Jacqueline then walked with us, and we got our bags and followed her to a vehicle waiting to take us to the hotel. I had never been to New York, so when I watched how the driver made it through the narrow streets with vehicles parked bumper-to-bumper and trash in piles on the curbside, I was amazed.

Jordan's Voice

The driver arrived at the hotel, and we took our bags and followed Jacqueline in to get our passkeys. Jacqueline then escorted us up to our room, and I gave her the memorial video and some pictures for their production department to get ready to use for the morning show. She then asked if we needed anything, and I said, "Can you direct us where to get something to drink and snack on till morning?" The free peanuts on the plane did not fill me up enough, and I usually like to have something to drink in the middle of the night. She showed us the convenience store at the corner. We thanked her and said, "We will see you in the morning." We headed to the store and picked up a few drinks and snacks, then headed back to our room and called for a 5:30 a.m. wake-up call and went to bed.

The morning came quickly, and even though we did not get a lot of sleep, we managed; I was used to getting up at 5:00 a.m. because of work. We showered and I shaved, and we then got dressed. Everything was ready, and we headed across the street to the studio. We met Jacqueline. We had to check in and receive temporary ID cards. As soon as we finished acquiring those, Jacqueline took us to the studio area, where I was prepped for the show with makeup. When they were through, they had me wait with my girlfriend in a room next to the studio until they were ready. Was I nervous? Yes, I was nervous, even though I knew I had to share my son's voice with everyone and let people know how I felt and wake up America to the fact there are things we can't ignore. Jacqueline received the call they were ready and for me and my girlfriend to follow her to the studio area. My girlfriend followed Jacqueline, and I followed another gentleman to a side stage with a couple of chairs and a table; they hooked a mic up to me, and Chris Cuomo came over and introduced himself and gave me his condolences for the loss of my son. He sat across from me and stated, "Look at me during the conversation." The cameraman gave him fifteen seconds, then Chris began to speak.

"Good morning. We have Brad Lewis, the father who poured his heart out with a YouTube video that went viral speaking out about bullying and how his son took his life over being bullied." Chris looked over to me and started asking questions about what happened when I first received the news and what was going through my mind that brought me to make the video.

I said, "I was in shock and didn't know really what to say. I was at work; I received a call from his mom, and then I called a zone lieutenant to come to my spot ASAP. They came, relieved me, and drove me home, but I was filled with so many emotions. Who knows what could have happened? My main thought, I guess, was to find out everything so this would not happen again to another child or parent losing their child." I know my eyes were beginning to water up, but I did the best I could.

Chris wrapped it up and thanked me for coming at short notice. Again, he stated he was sorry for my family's loss. I walked off the set and met my girlfriend and Jacqueline, and we headed back to get our coats. Jacqueline then took us into the broadcasting building to have breakfast, where we talked more about the incident and then had simple conversation. When we were finished, we walked back over to the hotel, and Jacqueline told us, "If you want to stay an extra day, you can; we will change your flight out for tomorrow morning." I turned and looked at my girlfriend and said, "You missed enough work because of Jordan's death." She asked Jacqueline if we could get an early morning flight out; she confirmed we could. So we agreed to stay one extra day, then Jacqueline said, "I will have a driver standing by in the morning for you to get to the airport."

We left the hotel and went on a walk in Times Square and surrounding areas, as well as to the Twin Towers memorial. I remember that day—9/11—very well. It was my birthday, and I was home from work, enjoying my day off and playing a game. I received a call and said, "Turn on the news." The first plane had already hit the first tower, then a few minutes went by, and the second plane hit the tower. It was an incredibly sad day for our country, but I had my own sadness to deal with. When we visited the Twin Towers memorial, there were cameras every fifteen yards apart, so they saw everything you did, then when you got farther in, they scanned you like they do at the airports before you could enter the memorial site. This was the final resting spot of every soul lost in 9/11, with all their names etched in stone as well. We also went into the cathedral by the Stock Exchange and marveled at how detailed this historical building was, then we headed back down the street to see all the buildings, going a different route until we made it back to Times Square. You could see the buildings where talk show hosts did their shows and all the lights and big signs. We had dinner there in Times Square and just watched the lights and people passing by.

I tried to enjoy it, even at the memorial, thinking how peaceful it was as the water flowed over the side into a large square hole. I was that hole at that moment, but I was not peaceful at all. I was tired, and my girlfriend said, "Let's head back to the room and get our stuff packed for tomorrow morning," since we had to leave super early to get to the airport. I checked my email and Facebook and noticed several responses, especially one from this lady named Beth who was so sorry for what had happened; she had messaged me a few days earlier and wanted to help us out. She stated that she did web design, God had spoken to her and her husband through the Holy Spirit, and she wanted to assist us.

CHAPTER EIGHT

I told my girlfriend, but I did not want to respond to Beth until I was back home and could focus more on things, because I still had to figure out the rest of the bills for Jordan's funeral and his headstone. Wow! All this, and it really had not started yet—I mean, getting Jordan buried and then wanting to find who, what, where, and why, as well as letting people know how serious this subject was.

There was nothing else to look at for the moment, so I shut down the computer, and we headed out for another walk to Times Square. We just walked, and it was amazing how the streets were just as busy in the evening, with people going to eat and catch shows. I like visiting places and seeing people active, but I love quiet places just as much—not dead, but quiet, a place not too far from activity, but somewhere where it is not too overpopulated and there is not someone living right on top of you. I remember the bike rides Jordan and I would take, riding from the bike hub where I lived all the way through Granite City up the river road to Alton and Grafton, where we would fill up our water bladders and ride back home, making it a seventy-three-mile trip. Jordan was proud of that because he could do it, and not many kids that age would even attempt it. He was tired, but he accomplished it, and I was proud of him as well.

My girlfriend asked if I was OK or if I needed to sit. I said, "No, I'm OK, just had some thoughts of me and Jordan, but I'm good." There was a big assortment of things to do, but we did not have the time to do them. We walked down to a pizza place, bought two slices of pizza and drinks, and walked back to the hotel. We were finished by the time we reached the hotel and went to our room; my feet were sore, so I jumped into the shower and got out, brushed my teeth, and took my meds, then called for a 3:00 a.m. wake-up and fell asleep.

The early morning came with a wake-up call, and we were up getting things together. I washed my face and brushed my teeth, and my girlfriend did the same. We got dressed and checked the room to make sure we had not left anything, then headed down to the lobby. We turned in our room key and headed outside, where the driver was standing by. We loaded up and took off to the airport. When we arrived, we said our goodbyes to Jacqueline and thanked her for her gracious assistance while we were there. She said Chris Cuomo was sending me a gift for coming on the show as well.

We hurried after getting there to get through the security checkpoints and grab a snack and drinks before boarding the plane. We waited for approximately twenty minutes before boarding. The view was a little different taking off this time, with a little bit of light on the horizon, but not much. The view was delightful, but I laid my head back and fell right to sleep before we got back to Saint Louis, where I would drop my girlfriend off at work. The plane arrived and taxied to the terminal. We unloaded and picked up our baggage, then caught a shuttle to my vehicle and headed out.

I dropped my girlfriend off at her work and drove home, staying there till I came back and picked her back up that evening; she came back to my house to pick her car up and went home to get some needed sleep. I needed sleep as well, because I was physically and mentally tired from everything from the past week. I know when I lay down in my bed, I tried crying, but there was no use—I was so worn out, I did not have the energy to. The next morning, I took my clothes from the trip down and placed them in the washer, then I fixed myself something to eat and headed back up to get on the computer. I started looking through my Facebook account and contacted Beth, who said she had already put together a website for my son and attached it to Facebook and gave me the password to control the domain. I looked over it and began seeing responses from people, but I also went back to my Facebook page to catch up with people leaving comments; there were a few. Most of them were stories from people about how they were bullied growing up, and others were parents who had kids who were being or had been bullied and the principal had done nothing to correct the situation. Then I read a message from a lady from my son's town. She began talking about being kindhearted and forgiving to the ones who had done the bullying, that they might come forward with answers, but if I continued telling public stories from others that she believed to be untrue, she would mention an order of protection I had from eleven and a half years prior. I gave my number to the lady and said, "Please call me, because you don't know what you're talking about." She replied, "OK."

About ten minutes later, I received a call from this lady. Her name was Biz! I say that with emphasis because you will realize what I mean when I am through. I asked Biz what the nature of the order of protection was, and she stated, "People make mistakes, and sure, they change, but they should be empathetic and forgiving as they were forgiven." I then stated, "Biz, the order of protection you're talking about came during the time me and my ex-wife were going through separation, and my son wanted to live with me." I then went on to tell her that when my kids and I went out to eat, she and her friend would come by the house and take things we had not agreed on. I explained, "I was tired of the games, and I was filing for divorce and wanted to let the court decide on where he lives. I dropped my son off at my parents' house to see my attorney. When I returned, she had come by and taken my son from my parents' house, and I found that she had an attorney file a temporary restraining order on me, which was dissolved two weeks later, because it was untrue. So there was no physical altercation between me and my ex-wife, ever." And then I said, "If there had been, I would not be able to possess a concealed weapons card or work for corrections. Since there was no validity to the order of protection, all you're doing is trying to defame my character as a person."

She then said, "I just want you to see the school already stated there was no official documentation of bullying." I could not believe this lady wanted to intimidate and threaten me. Was she acting on her own because her child could have been involved, or was she the community busybody? I finished talking to her and began calling the state attorney's office and the sheriff's office to talk to the lead detective, who sent me an email of my son's suicide note. I read the note. It was hard for me to read. It was as if he felt there was no way out and life was not going to get any better. I cried! I cried because it hurt me to know how much he had to be hurting to do this and think this world would be better off without him. The anger grew inside of me, and then I was messaged by a few parents on Facebook asking if I was going to attend the school board meeting the next Monday or Tuesday, because there were several parents wanting answers to what had happened. I said I might be there to hear what they had to say.

I decided to call the superintendent and let him know I would be showing up with other parents, wanting to hear what their views were. When I talked to the superintendent, I asked if he had viewed the anti-bullying video that was shown on October 16, 2013, at the school. The superintendent replied no, he had not. So I stated, "How can you show something that you or the principal have never viewed before to children and not even contact their parents and get their permission to view the video?" I told him I would be at the meeting, but he stated he would rather I come to his office for a private meeting with him and a few school board members and discuss this matter discreetly. I said, "There are other parents with issues themselves that want to ask questions and have concerns." The superintendent's reply was, "They can schedule private meetings as well, separately, and we can deal with them, but I would prefer not doing this at the school board meeting." Then he said, "The board meeting is scheduled in advance to discuss the school's financial status and where best to spend money and cut money for the upcoming year." I stated, "There are several parents who are coming to the meeting, and I knew nothing about it until one parent messaged me about it." The superintendent still insisted that I and the other parents did not need to come to the meeting, that this could be managed behind closed doors. I said, "Sorry, sir, but I can't control other people on how they feel."

The conversation was over. I was done talking and aggravated with the idea he wanted no one to hear about what was going to be said, so it would be their word against mine. Wow! What else would I have to deal with trying to find out the whole truth? I knew why they were hiding what happened. The reason was the status of their community, funding, and politics with the election year right around the corner. The thing is, it was a sad situation, putting prestige and money over the safety and well-being of the children in the community because your school and community might lose social status. The rest of the day, I was talking to Beth; she had Jordan's website put together and had the CNN interview already posted on the site and was getting a Facebook page going as well. She initially had it flowing through my daughter's Facebook page, but my girlfriend mentioned to me that it should be independent so people could contact me and there were no missed communications about what I was trying to get accomplished. So Beth changed the Facebook page for Jordan's Voice to be independent so it could be tied to my Facebook page.

I sat back after getting off my computer and just started thinking about when I was little, dealing with bullying and the impact it had on me then and later in life. I mean, I went sixteen years without being bullied or harassed, and as a grown man, I became a victim of bullying and harassment at my job. The thing is, I was in a hostile environment already, dealing with the worst of the worst in a prison setting, but then I was harassed daily—whether in a cell house or in a tower, they would find a way. You might ask, how can they harass you in a tower? One, the ringer—they would constantly call you, let it ring, and when you answered, hang up on you. Now, it was not the same one; they would have guys from other towers, or another cell house call you until you unhooked your phone. That was at the old institution, but the new facility was finding ways to keep me from getting promoted, and that became a management issue. So I thought, "Why am I still alive and not Jordan? What was so important that I am still here and not my little buddy?" I talked to and prayed to God so much to guide me and give me the strength to figure this out and help me make something positive from this for Jordan's sake.

The next morning, I woke up early as usual to call into work for a day off and went back to sleep. I would sleep until eight or nine and try to get myself out of bed and fix myself something to eat and bring it back up to my room. I would then turn on the television for background noise and get on my computer to check the Facebook accounts and view the comments from children and parents on the status of bullying or comments on things going on in my son's school district. There were several people messaging me about the school board meeting as well as Channel 3 and Channel 12 news being there to talk to me before the meeting and being there as well. Then I heard about a boy in Nevada who had gone to school the next day after viewing a similar movie at his school about bullying and shot and killed the kids who bullied him and a teacher trying to protect the boys. The child then took the gun and shot himself, committing suicide, showing he accomplished what he had set out to do, and that was to punish the bullies and end his suffering at the cost of an innocent man's life, that of the teacher. I was angry, because kids who are bullied do not understand that their actions have short-term effects and long-term ones as well. They think it is fun, or "Who cares," but the loss of a person's life may influence any number of other people, and then that individual who bullied will have to carry the burden of their actions the rest of their lives.

I received calls from the *LA Times* and other papers requesting phone interviews and one from a college paper; the reporter wanted to meet me at the school meeting when I came down. I was keeping busy with the phone calls and scheduling to meet with people to tell Jordan's story. I stopped and started thinking about that night, because Jordan and I had tickets for the Eagles concert in Saint Louis, and I had no way to sell them to anyone because they cost so much. I was going to go with my girlfriend so I could get out and relax to some good music, but my thoughts of Jordan kept flowing, and I stepped into his room and laid on his bed, tears rolling down my cheeks. I was remembering all the fun times he and I'd had horsing around. I would get him down, tickling him until he would yell, "Uncle! I have to go pee." Then he would laugh, running out of the room, saying, "I was kidding," then run into the bathroom.

My girlfriend finally talked me into going to the concert. So I started picking things up and putting them away and organizing all the papers, notes, and sticky notes with people's names. I was finished getting ready and just waiting for my girlfriend to arrive. As soon as she did, she came in and changed, and then we headed out to the Scottrade Center. I am always good at being somewhere ahead of time—something the military had instilled in me. We hurried and found a good parking spot, then walked across the street to the concert venue. The thing about getting somewhere early is that you stand in line and meet people you would never expect to, but I was not too much into talking at all that evening. They finally let us go in, and we found our way to the promotion booth where they sold their items. I bought a shirt as I usually do, and from there, we found the restrooms and used them. When we came out, we purchased drinks and snacks and headed to our seats.

The last time Jordan and I were at the Scottrade Center, we were on the main floor and had to stand the whole concert, and my legs were very sore by the end of the evening. That was the Bon Jovi concert, and Jordan had a blast; he was enjoying the music that evening and dancing with the rhythm of the music. Even though my girlfriend was with me this night, it was not the same; Jordan and I had a bond in which we enjoyed going to concerts, games, and movies and would goof off and aggravate each other as well.

The people started slowly filling the seats. We made a move to use the restrooms again before the band started and returned to our seats. We settled in, and then the lights dimmed. The spotlight set on one member as he would talk, and then another would come out, then they would play a song to introduce another member. This continued until they had introduced all the band members, and then they started playing as a total band. The music was good, but my girlfriend would look over and ask if I was OK. It was hard as I sat back with my eyes full of tears, trying to hold them back. It was difficult for songs being played that he and I would sing to while we drove back to my place, or I took him home. My chest was hurting as if I were having a heart attack, and then I would take a deep breath and rub my chest.

My girlfriend looked over and asked if I was all right again. I just said, "Yes, it's just the pain of missing him." Tears were rolling down my cheeks. I added, "I need to use the restroom." Quickly, I jumped up and headed to the restroom and used the facilities; when finished, I walked over to the sink and splashed water in my face and cleared my eyes, then wiped my face with a paper towel. I took a moment, then took a couple of deep breaths and went back and sat down and listened to the rest of the concert.

We started heading out when they began doing an encore song; we listened as we made our way around the outer hall to the entrance through which we had come in. The drive home was quiet. I did say the music was good, but maybe not worth the cost of the tickets. It was not as good because I was thinking about Jordan, and when you have something like that on your mind, then it is hard to really enjoy much of anything. We headed back to my place. She went home, and I showered and went to bed, but before going to sleep, I said a prayer. I thanked God for everything and told him how much I hurt from missing my son and asked if he would guide me every day to make the right choices to spread Jordan's voice as best as I could. Then I fell asleep.

The next morning, I woke up and laid in bed for a short while, then I greeted the morning, saying, "Good morning, God, Jesus, Jordan, Dad, and Little Roger in heaven." Then I rolled out of bed and into the bathroom to shock myself with a quick cold shower and then a warm shower for the stiffness in my knees and my back. Every day, I had to wake up early and call work to let them know I was taking another day off instead of saying I would not be returning till a certain time; that is how my work did things. I started heading downstairs to get something to eat, then I looked at my phone. I had several messages from Beth, the web designer, telling me to call her, asking me about things and what we should be focusing on. She told me she had an idea about something, and the Holy Spirit had directed her to do this for Jordan's cause. I was awake and I gave her a call, but she fired at me with both barrels a-blazing, asking who I was interviewed by and when my next interview was, saying we needed to get fired up for the Bears versus Rams game. I really appreciated her help, but so much was hitting me at one time, I needed to step back to see everything. Sometimes it is hard to manage so many aspects of something, and with Beth, I had to make sure she was making choices in my son's best interest. Sometimes she would criticize someone posting on the website and would say, "That person's website is too violent," or, "This one is nonreligious," and if someone who was gay supported Jordan's Voice, she did not want them commenting or being friends on this site because it did not represent her beliefs. I went along with her only because she was doing it for free and because I had no real direction yet except hoping for a positive outcome to keep this from ever happening again.

When I was done with Beth, my girlfriend called asking me how everything was then commenting on what some people were saying on Facebook and telling me about what Ms. Biz was saying as well. As you will remember, Ms. Biz is the lady that was trying to threaten me if I did not stop all this, the busybody of my son's community. I then called the lead detective and asked for a clearer copy of my son's suicide note and sent him all the emails from the parents and kids of that community so he could contact them and take statements from them. He responded that he would investigate them, but if the kids did not come in and give statements, he could not do anything about it. I asked, "Are you going to confiscate my son's computer, cell phone, and iPod to see if anything is on there I did not know about?"

When I was through talking to the detective, I started making calls, calling even the White House. A certified letter had to be sent to them. Then I received a text message from Beth saying, "Hi, Brad! This is where we're at, and can you type something explaining how you are feeling each day and how it is affecting you with Jordan's passing and how much you miss him as well?" She went on, "We have to keep the page flowing and keep people's attention on what's going on, or we will lose people's interest." I did not want a stock report every day; I wanted people to be able to go to the page and tell what they knew about the issues at my son's school and what they knew about Jordan. Then I wanted children and parents from across the country to share their stories of how they had been dealing with bullying in their schools and whether the schools were managing it or not doing anything at all. There are a lot of stories out there, and I wanted people to express with honesty their situations so other children knew they were not alone and that if we stand together for the same cause, we can get everyone to stop, look, and listen about the problems at hand.

I read a story—I believe it was about a community in a state near our state. A girl was raped by a player on the football team at a party. The mother went to the school and complained. Nothing was done, so she got an attorney, and it became public. The town turned on them and went and burned their house down. That was negative support for the girl who was raped, who was humiliated, with her family treated like outcasts. I know there are communities that are out there like that in some way or another—they may not burn your house, but they will politically burn you and your reputation. That means keeping you from getting job advancements or financial loans, which ends up keeping your family financially down and sometimes causes you to lose everything, including your family and marriage. I know because I have talked to people who would not give their names due to possible repercussions from their kids' school system or the chance the community might ignore them completely. The important thing is, parents think that they have argued with schoolteachers and administrators, and nothing has been done, so their children suffer mental and physical abuse not just from other kids but sometimes from the faculty. This does not mean all faculty are like that; I have talked to schoolteachers who have said their hands are tied, depending on who the kid is and how important he is to the school.

Well, as the day went on into the evening, my girlfriend called and said that she was leaving work and would stop by. Throughout the evening, Beth was instant messaging me on Facebook, asking questions, and she was texting my girlfriend throughout the day, asking her what she thought about things, or she was communicating with my daughter Deeanna about how she was dealing with things, telling her she needed to delete certain people from her site because they did not represent the right type of people for Jordan's Voice against Bullying. So we told my daughter to be careful of responding to people who reached out to her, because some people prey on others' hardships so they can gain a profit or get themselves connected with other people you know to exploit your site for their own benefit. The day was ending, and my girlfriend asked if I wanted to do anything like get a bite to eat or watch a movie; we headed out and went to the movies just to get out of my apartment and move around and breathe. While we were out at the movie, Beth was messaging me and texting, asking if I was busy and could get online. I said I was not home, that I was at the movies. She said, "OK. I need to get with you so we can get more things flowing on the website, and I need your attention as soon as possible." I texted back that I would get ahold of her as soon as I got home that evening. I really do not recall the movie, because it was only a slight distraction from what was really happening around me. I received a few more text messages from Beth, as did my girlfriend, but my girlfriend was able to text back and let her know we were at the movies, and we would get back to her when we got home.

When the show was over, we headed back to my place and then contacted Beth. She answered, and we exchanged information so she could get more info out on the web page and discuss programs I wanted to do or even interviews I had done so she could load them to the website and Facebook page. I gave Jordan's site its name because so many people use justice for this or that, and I knew when I told her the name, she would say, "No, it sounds too vengeful." The next thing that came to my mind was hearing my son's voice again, so I said, "Jordan's Voice against Bullying." She agreed, and that would be his signature. I now look back at when I helped a boy with developmental problems, and I did a fundraiser to get him a second wish since he lived longer than a lot of people expected.

CHAPTER NINE

Every child deserves a chance to go to school and learn without having to worry about being picked on before or after school and not having to go online and see stuff posted about them that keeps them from keeping their eye on the ball. Quality of life is what we all deserve, not just in school but when we grow up as well. Workplace harassment is more common than we think, and many things develop from people being bullied or even harassed at work. Life is not a fairy tale or a movie, and many times, it is plain ugly. Why?

We see every day all the ugliness around us, but do we do anything about it? *No.* We continue to listen to and believe the same old lies that are fed to us, and we then ignore what is really going on. I told Beth that I was heading to bed and to post about the school board meeting that coming Monday to rally people to attend. My girlfriend headed home because I was tired, worn out, and ready to head to bed; I needed some time for my mind to reboot. So much was happening so soon, and I had the school board meeting and interviews to think about so I could get a clear picture to the nation, instructing them about what to really look at. The behavior of students reflects how the administration deals with children who have issues treating other children properly; if the teachers and administration do not stand up for the kids being bullied and continue to allow it, then the problem gets worse. I look back and remember how teachers placed me in the corner, the clothes closet, or in the hallway because I was supposedly a distraction to them, when really, they were distracting me, and I could not focus and learn properly the way I should have.

My girlfriend left, and I walked back into my room, taking my medicine and saying my prayers, asking God to give me strength to assist me in getting the word out on the safety and well-being of the children and to tell my son I loved and missed him. Saturday morning came, and I laid in bed for a bit before I jumped up and took a shower. After my morning routine, I went downstairs and grabbed something to drink, then went back to my room and turned on my television and computer. I started the morning reviewing Jordan's Facebook page and website to check the responses and to respond to people who had things to say; I saw the responses in which kids and others said their goodbyes and expressed that they missed him. I sat back in my chair, saying, "Why him? Why would someone bully such a good boy who only wants to be friends and be a part of something and make people laugh in his own way?" Tears rolled down my cheeks as I looked at pictures of him, still remembering the good times and thinking about what he would be like after graduating high school and going into the army and then college.

Plus, he never really had a chance to be part of his brother's and sister's lives, even when they lived so close to him. Jordan's mom used him as a pawn, and even though my parents would pick him up and bring him to their house so his siblings could see him, his mom would not let him. Jordan loved them and his grandpa and grandma on my side of the family, which is why he wanted to be buried by his Grandpa Lewis. Jordan mentioned in his suicide note that before my dad (Grandpa Lewis) died, "I saw grandpa lying in his bed a few weeks before dying and I saw God standing by his side." I think he saw Jesus standing by his side taking care of him. So, as he mentioned, he wanted to be buried where there was a spot for him, and he knew there were two plots left by Grandpa Lewis.

I was not mad at God; I knew Satan had taken a part of my soul to discourage me from growing closer to God. Many say they are a good Christian because they go to church twice a week and put money into the offering plate. I do not, but that does not mean God hates me for it. When I was younger, I went to church all the time, but when we moved down south away from Chicago, I became a teenager and played sports, fished at the lake, and went to the movies on the weekends. I became too busy to go and drifted away from God, and that was my excuse for drifting away. I tried going back repeatedly, especially down in the town I grew up in, but I was not part of their socioeconomic clique. I even found that one of my good friends never even came to my son's funeral, though his mom did. There were several people I went to school with who distanced themselves from me because they lived in that county, and they did not want any negative repercussions coming back on them for supporting my cause. Politics is the best way to describe some of it; another way is not trying to do the right thing when the right thing is what is needed.

Satan had been discouraging me for years, and God has always been there to pick me up, no matter what. I have read the Bible and many other spiritual books by religious authors, and I research the info in the Bible online as well. So I did speak to Jordan about God and how he needed to read his Bible and pray to him at night or in the day silently in his mind so no one knew what he was saying except for God, because he knows what is on your mind. Jordan knew where I stood; I would always ask him, "Have you been reading your Bible or praying at night?" I gave Jordan a book to read: *Revelation Unveiled*, by Tim LaHaye. It broke down the Book of Revelation so a child could understand it and explained what the end days were going to be like when Jesus returned. Jordan read all of it, and one weekend, when he came to visit, he asked me how to be saved. I sat down with my son and went through a prayer with him. I said, "Son, you have to admit to God you're a sinner and that you accept Jesus Christ as your Lord and Savior and that he died on the cross for your sins so that you can live eternal life through the blood that he shed on that cross of Calvary." Jordan understood and accepted Christ that day. I was proud, because I knew he wanted to go to church, but his mother would never let him.

I got back to my computer, reading more stories from people, and as I was reading them, Beth noticed I was online and messaged me right away. "We need to do this before the meeting." I replied, "What?" She explained, "You need to figure out what your long-term goal and focus on Jordan's Voice is." Then the topic of a foundation came up, and she asked whether I would consider this option. I said, "I do not know. All this happened eight or nine days ago. I would like for something positive to come out of this, even if we could join up with a larger foundation—that might be better." She was not in favor of that. "No. You never know when another entity might do something wrong and bring your group down with them."

I knew that I could focus on only so much at a time, and even for my girlfriend, it started to feel like a lot of drama with Beth constantly texting and messaging her. Beth even made my girlfriend an administrator on the site so she could help observe the posts and if people were coming online to bully others, remove them. I know my son's mom's sister would get on there and ask, "Who oversees this app, and why are comments removed?" They would reply, "We are the administrator for the father, and we try and keep things peaceful." His mother would never say anything but instead have someone else do it. Jordan's mom never spoke up about his suicide and would never do an interview, and when I asked her for Jordan's computer, which I had bought him, she said, "I tried getting on it and took it to a computer person I know, and he said the drive was fried." I knew that was a lie, because I had just had everything looked over by the Best Buy Geek Squad and put a new Webroot program on his system and had his drive decompressed; it was just like new. I figured Jordan had things that would point fingers, and she did not want me to get ahold of it and had someone do something to it, so she never gave it back to me. Then when I met her and her best friend so she could give me the last child support check and some things of his, she blamed me for his death and said, "I should have fought harder for him. If I had, he might be alive."

I was like, "How is it my fault? When he was younger, in fourth and fifth grade, he ran away from you when you lived across the state, trying to get to my house. And the first time he called me from a gas station, and I had to call the cops and let them know where he was. The second time he was trying to come to my house, he ducked down in a ditch to avoid being seen by you and got stuck in a tree root, and luckily, you found him. When I asked if he could come and stay with me until we figured things out, your response was, 'I would have him placed in juvenile detention before I would allow him to live with you.'"

I kept copies of the police reports so I could keep them at hand in case something happened again. I told Beth I might investigate stronger guidelines within the state and see if that would work, but for now, I needed some me time, and I would get back to her. My girlfriend came over and wanted to get me out of the apartment to grab a bite to eat or drive over to Soulard Market in Saint Louis and pick up a few items, then get something to eat over there. When we were finished, we came back to my place and I told her I was going to relax and spend time by myself. It was not that I didn't want to spend time with her, but I needed time to think and pray about things. She was all right with that and headed home.

Sunday morning came, and I was lying in bed, deciding what I was going to do and when I was going to get myself out of bed. I knew the school board meeting was the coming Tuesday and that I would be driving down to my son's town for it. What I would say and how I would manage myself were the real questions. I asked God to give me answers so I could go in levelheaded, even though I knew they were going to brush me off. I finally found the energy to get myself out of bed, taking myself downstairs to the kitchen to get some juice and make some egg whites to eat. I then positioned myself back in my room at my desk in front of my computer and turned on the television to hear the news. I went back and forth, reviewing comments and reading articles and then taking a break to watch something—news, cartoons, or a movie. Still, throughout the day, Beth would text me and say, "You need to put a comment out to keep things moving to get people to respond and get outside interaction from the public." I did not know how his mom was feeling, because she had to live with the thought that the police were there the night before at her home doing a wellness check on Jordan; as you will remember, a call had come in saying he commented to someone he was going to kill himself. No one calls the police and reports that someone wants to hurt themselves unless they feel it is a legitimate threat. Him telling that girl he was going to do this was him reaching out for help, and only one girl took him seriously and told her grandmother, whom she lived with. The day gradually moved on, and I then got out of my chair and showered, signed off Facebook, took my sleep medicine, said my prayers, and told Monkey Butt good night.

Monday was just another day like most since Jordan's death. It is hard to keep track of everything that has happened, so most of the rest of the book will be the main things I have talked about and what has happened or what was said or done in meetings or interviews. A person can only remember so much unless they keep a tape recorder or a notebook to keep track or have a photographic memory of things they have seen or heard.

Tuesday morning, I was up early, showered and dressed, put things in the jeep, then headed off to my sister's house. I gassed up, grabbed something to drink and a breakfast sandwich, and headed on my way. I had already scheduled interviews with three news media outlets and a phone interview with the college paper that all had to be done before going to the school board meeting that evening. The main thing was to state what I knew and the problem, even though the superintendent did not want me to be present and asked if other parents and I would meet with him and a couple other school board members quietly; I could not do that. Doing it their way would make it about their statements versus mine, and I wanted everyone to hear what their responses were to my questions. I know among the reasons for them to do it their way instead of mine was to keep me quiet, along with deniability and damage control, so their community looked good, and they had no issues in their schools. Reminds me of the Penn State incident—you know things are happening, but you just turn your head and ignore the issue at hand and hope no one knows the truth.

I have already told you that Jordan loved to be a part of things, even sports, even though he wasn't good. He played his freshman year in football and was a special team player; he had issues with some players, and there was that incident where the kid punched him in the back of the head for no reason. His sophomore year, he went to summer practices before school started, and when school began, he heard there was a one-day golf tryout. He asked the football coach if he could try out for the golf team and if he did not make it, to go to football practice the next day. The football coach said, "If you don't go to practice today, you're not playing." Jordan went to try out for golf, since it was kind of an individual sport, and he thought he might not get picked on while playing. Well, he didn't make it, and the next day, he tried to go to football practice, and the coach said no.

I arrived in town and first stopped off at Jordan's grave and spoke to him in my own way, asking God to give me the strength to do this. I then proceeded to the places I needed to go for the interviews. I spoke to each person. I was trying to keep myself together, but one lady asked me, "If Jordan were here, what would you say to him if you were able to talk to him one more time?" I nearly lost it. Now, I do not know what kept me together. But yes, I do know! God was my strength, holding me together even though my heart was broken; his love kept me strong. Then, after finishing the interviews, I had to get something to eat, and so I stopped at the nearest fast-food place to grab a bite. I had to meet one more newsperson outside of the school before the school board meeting, so I had to rush and get my food down and get there. I was mentally tired and still had a few more hours to endure at the meeting.

I arrived at the school and parked in the parking lot by the rear entrance near the auditorium. When I got out, I noticed the reporter by her vehicle. I walked up and introduced myself, and she began setting up her equipment. Once she was finished, she told me to relax and explained what she was going to ask in general. I took a deep breath and waited for her questions, and I answered each question with a simple reply to the best I could. The interview was done, and I noticed a few police officers walking into the school. Just then, my mom, brother, and sister pulled up. I walked up to them and hugged them. We walked in together; as we walked into the auditorium, there were three police officers from the town in there in full gear and body armor except for the helmet. I walked up to one and asked if it was normal for a school board meeting to have three police officers attending. The officer replied, "We're at all functions." I just smiled and said, "OK."

We found a seat, and a few people came up to me and gave their condolences, saying how sorry they were about what happened. The meeting started. There were three camera crews from different stations present and filming. The superintendent started his presentation, and as he went along, all he was talking about was how great their school district was and how much their property was worth. He then patted himself on the back, stating their school was one of the top ten schools in the state. I could not stand it. I raised my hand, and he refused to acknowledge me. Then I spoke up and said, "Mr. Superintendent, how about the safety and well-being of the children—is that worth more than your property?"

He still ignored me; one of the officers walked up behind me and touched me on the shoulder, then said, "Mr. Lewis, you will have your time to speak. Just ignore it and let him speak; I know you're upset." I do not know what kind of emotion you could have placed on me to describe how I was feeling. He just stood up there and smiled while speaking to the audience. "We need to figure out how to spend the extra ten percent if we have it and where we can cut ten percent if the government does not give us the money." He continued to brag about their new junior high and high school and the fact that they had the best football field in the whole southern region, repeating that their property was worth about $160 million and adding they would like to build a new administration building for him and his faculty. At no time did the superintendent bring up anything about my son's death or that there could be an issue for them to investigate; that would have just opened the door to the fact they knew about bullying issues and had ignored the problem.

The superintendent said, "Everyone will break up into separate groups based on the color circle on your handout." So as soon as he concluded, we divided up into subgroups in different classrooms so no one could hear what I had to say. The camera crew followed me, and I found a spot in the back of the room. Then, lo and behold, in steps the superintendent. Separating everyone had been planned, and I was sure the people that were in my classroom were people he had handpicked. He then asked me what I was going to say in front of the camera so he could act concerned about my son, but he was not concerned. The man never said a word to me thereafter; I refused to tell him what I was going to say, and he never mentioned anything about how to improve the situation of bullying in the school. There were numerous responses to other ideas, and a few people did mention the safety and well-being of the children in the school. Then a few said, "An extra language class would be good."

The meeting was finished, and my family and I began to head out. One of the officers told me that they never attend school board meetings, and that the superintendent requested their presence. We left the building, and I hugged my family goodbye. My mom asked, "Son, are you OK to drive back home? You can stay the night with Mom." I replied, "I'm good, Mom," and left. During my drive back, I talked to God, and then I was thinking of what I could do to make it safer for kids so this would not happen to any other children, and they would not have to suffer as Jordan did. The drive back was good, but I had Beth texting me asking how everything was and what stations and papers interviewed me so she could look them up and post them to Jordan's website. I made it home, undressed, and stepped into a warm shower, enjoying the heat on my body; it relaxed my sore, tired muscles and joints. I dried off, took my sleeping meds, put my shorts and T-shirt on, and hopped into bed, then fell fast asleep after saying my prayers.

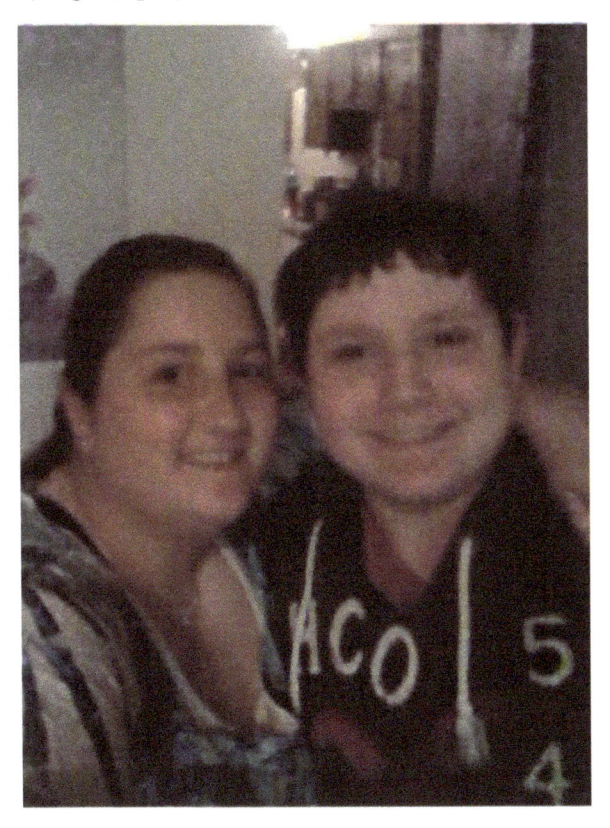

CHAPTER TEN

Every morning since Jordan's death, I would wake up hoping it was all a nightmare and that I would hear his voice or know I would see him on the weekend when we had things planned. The only problem was it was real! I had to drag myself out of bed; even if it was just to the shower or my desk, the amount of energy used to get me to either place was a lot. Like I said before, I cannot remember everything I did, but I was going to prepare for the school board meeting, which was coming up in November. I was supposed to return to work on November 4 and face the people and the inmates. Well, I worked the rest of the week, preparing things I wanted to focus on in terms of changes, reading articles, replying to people on Jordan's Facebook page, and preparing for the November 17 Bears versus Rams game in Saint Louis, which I had purchased tickets for me and Jordan to go to. Beth, the web designer, was busy preparing info on the game to rally people for the occasion, but it seemed like each week, she was pushing me to commit to a foundation and getting too involved with personal business involving my daughter and my girlfriend—having conversations in which she told them what to post on their Facebook sites and then telling me what I needed to focus on and pushing other things aside, even my relationship. I know people want to give their advice or input, but I already had Biz butting into my life, telling me I was not telling the exact truth and threatening me so I would back off what I was doing, or she would expose my order of protection to the world. So, I had a person threatening and trying to intimidate me during a time I was fighting back after my son took his life due to bullying by kids in the same town my son lived in.

Jordan's Voice

I worked during the days before the next meeting, writing things for the Jordan's Voice Facebook page, trying to reach out to people and educate them about how serious this problem really was. I had a sign business create a banner and yard sign; it was costly even though he took some of the price off. I even went and had business cards made at another place so that I could give people an opportunity to view Jordan's Facebook site and website.

November 4 came. I had to return to work, and everyone told me how sorry they were. I went through the workday as if it were just another day because the next day was what I was focusing on. I went to work on Tuesday and still did what needed to be done; I even had inmates who had seen the interviews or read the articles walk up to me and say they were sorry. I would say thank you, but I could not discuss it with them, and they understood. I was focused on getting off work and heading down to the school board meeting to hear if they were going to do anything or take the matter seriously.

I got out of work and began my drive. My thoughts were running rapid with ideas like Mel Gibson in the movie *Conspiracy Theory*. The county my son had lived in and the surrounding counties were very political, and keeping things quiet was their priority so their social status was not dragged through the mud. I prayed while driving, talking to God, but you know, it was not praying; I was talking to God as if I were having a regular conversation. I know he did not speak back to me like he did his prophets, but he was there to listen to me. I stopped and grabbed a sandwich and a soda as I passed through one of the towns before getting to my destination. As I got closer, I called my mom to let her know I was there.

I arrived. There were fewer cars there, but I was early, and so I headed in. I saw an officer walking in the student dietary area and walked toward him to ask where the meeting was; the auditorium was locked, so I was wondering if they had changed the dates. I approached the officer and asked if the meeting was still on. He said yes. I then asked him why they had officers at the meetings but not during the school day while school was in session. The officer replied, "We told them we would put in a grant for a resource officer to be there, but they replied that they had no need for one and it intimidated the students and made them feel threatened." He added, "I even told them I would walk the halls if they would fill out the federal grant form." I thanked the officer and headed back to the rear entrance, then waited for my mom and sister.

There were a few parents there about issues with their kids being bullied who said the schools had never done anything. One woman said she was told by the principal that she needed to quit babying her children and they needed to grow thicker skin. Then another woman had an incident with her son, who was a special needs student, telling a girl she was pretty; the girl felt weird about it and said something to the principal. The principal then followed the boy around in the lunch communal area with an old-style megaphone, yelling at the boy, "Do I look pretty? Does my wife look pretty? Does my daughter look pretty?" in front of the other kids. Then there was another incident with a boy; he was trying to get a petition signed by other students to try and get my son Jordan's football jersey number from his freshman year retired. The principal walked up to the boy and tried taking it away, because they were not going to consider it. How do you think I felt? I was dealing with individuals who thought they were the untouchables, especially since we had a state attorney who lived in the town and who had been in his position for twenty years and a state representative who lived in town and had been in office for three terms.

My mom and sister arrived, and we walked into the room where the board meeting was to take place. I noticed outside the room in the communal area of the lunchroom there were three uniformed officers as before. Wow! I felt as if I were an inmate on death row being followed by officers who were keeping an eye on me. We walked in and found a seat, then I noticed Jordan's mom's best friend was a couple of rows in front of me. The meeting came to order, and the board began their dialogue about who was present and what was on the agenda, then asked if there were any new concerns. During the meeting, Jordan's mom's best friend made a comment about how Jordan's mom read through all of his text messages and emails and that it was hard, but if kids did pick on him, we should forgive and remember that there are consequences to our actions; she added that her son was on the football team, and he had never had a problem, and she felt their community was great. What should I have expected from her? Jordan's mom did not want to show her face, and she said that she tried going through Jordan's computer but could not, but she had lied. During this whole time, Jordan's mom would not say anything, because she was worried about herself and not about her son and how he suffered. Jordan knew she would not believe him, and she would ignore it.

The board members thanked her for her comments, then my mother made a comment and so did my sister, but they did not give them the same credit as the friend of Jordan's mom. I felt like I could explode given how they responded to my mom's comments; I knew how my mother felt after losing a child three years before I was born. I said my piece, even though it did not matter to them. I was blowing hot air and would have been better off talking to the wall or arguing with myself in a mirror. By saying that, I mean the wall just stands there, no mind, and if I had argued with myself in a mirror, I could at least have given myself a good response or said I was sorry. They just looked dumbfounded and said much of nothing again, knowing their response could have legal ramifications. My eyes were filled with tears, but I did not let one fall and held them back.

When the meeting was over, I walked into the communal lunch area, where I said goodbye to the lady that had told me about her children being bullied. She said, "I will see you at the next meeting," and I replied, "No, I won't be there, because I have to work, and the drive after work there and back home is rough after getting up at 5:00 a.m. and working all day. This next meeting is yours." A reporter from the *Southern* newspaper spoke with me for a minute and then we headed out the door. I gave my mom and sister a hug and said goodbye before heading home and getting rested up before work the next morning. I had my talk with God on my drive home, and I spoke to my son Jordan. I was not expecting a response, but if an angel had appeared by my side and spoken with me, then my heart would have been at ease. Many things were going through my mind, and I was wondering if I would be able to do this on my own. I made it home safely and called my mom to let her know I had made it back, as she had asked me to do. I changed, took my meds, said my prayers, and went to sleep.

The next few weeks consisted of getting things together for the Bears versus Rams football game in Saint Louis. I was putting together a petition that Beth helped format; I gave her all that I wanted to accomplish on a proposal for a bill. Beth put some ads on the webpage asking people to wear blue and orange on the day of the game. Let us represent Jordan and his favorite football team! But also, I was going to put up his banner and walk around and get the petition signed by people to support the antibullying proposal, and I wanted it to be on the federal level. The proposal was to mandate that all states follow the guidelines of this proposal; further, if the states had a bill, it would mandate that they enforce their bill. Then sometime during the next five days, I received a call from Tad Brown, an attorney out of a firm in the county I lived in called George and Brown. They contacted me by email and wanted to represent Jordan's and my cause. I told him I had not contacted them, and it was Beth, the lady who did the website, that contacted them, acting like she was me. He said, "No, we have been watching the interviews and reading the articles in the paper and following your story in the media, and we would like to represent you." I was overwhelmed and did not know what to say, so I replied, "Sir, I have no money to retain or pay for an attorney." The attorney replied, "We are not asking for a payment unless we win your case, but we would meet first and ask that you bring everything you can and your Facebook messages from other parents and kids who have replied to you."

We made an appointment for me to come in on November 15 after I got off work. I was happy that someone was going to assist me in making positive changes and that Jordan's death would not be in vain. There are so many children, I have come to find, who have taken their lives or hurt themselves due to bullying, and people ignore it as it is something that has been going on for years. The point was to stop it, and if I could not stop it, then I would at least try and get the word out to save children's lives. November 15 arrived, and I got up that morning and began getting ready for work, putting my uniform on and making sure I had everything the attorney wanted. I went to work and completed my day as usual, left work, and headed over to the attorney's office for the meeting. I arrived, went to the receptionist to check in, and sat waiting until I was called in.

Jordan's Voice

I waited about ten minutes, then Tad Brown and his assistant walked up and greeted me. I returned the greeting and followed them to a conference room, where we sat down and began discussing everything.

While we were sitting there, I realized I knew Tad and asked, "Didn't you go to school with me?" and he replied, "Yes, I was a freshman when you were a senior." He added, "I have a lot involved in this as well; my niece and nephew live in the school district your son was in, and I don't want this happening to them either." Then he asked me what happened from my last conversation with Jordan during my weekend with him till the morning he took his life and I received the call from his mom at work. We covered a lot of information quickly. They received access to my Facebook page and his website, then we talked by conference call to another attorney that would be working on the case and concluded by signing the papers on the agreement and their fee if they won.

Tad stated, "We will have my assistant get back with you on any more information if needed," then asked if I was going to the next school board meeting the following Tuesday. I responded I wasn't planning on it since I went to the first two after Jordan's death. Tad said, "If you did, we would like to be there to overhear what they have to say or how they respond to your questions." I agreed to go the following Tuesday after work. I left the office feeling good that something was going to be done, but I remembered he said this would not be a quick case, and it could go on for a year or two.

I prayed to God on my drive back home and thanked him for sending representation to guide me, help me, and take some of this stress off me so I could get funds together to pay the funeral costs the insurance wasn't able to cover and for Jordan's headstone. Now I had to focus on Sunday and what I was going to be doing at the Bears versus Rams football game in Saint Louis—making sure I had enough petitions for people to sign and clipboards and pens as well. I signed onto Facebook Saturday letting everyone know and reminding them to focus on Jordan's team, "Da Bears." I remember a Chicago Bears hat Jordan wanted. I bought it, and he wanted a nickname embroidered on it: JDawg. He loved it; he was cool now, LOL. I sat there at my monitor just thinking of what he would have achieved if he had been allowed to grow up and go into the military to get his college money and what he would have studied. I know some people think that you can get through things like this, but I knew when I looked at my mom that my son's death had brought so many hard memories that she had overcome and dealt with; her seeing her baby boy lose his baby boy just about tore her into pieces all over again. Sometimes it is extremely hard for a person to get over a loss in their lives. Some do not, and it drives them to the grave as well.

Sunday came, and I was up and ready to head out. I wore my Walter Payton jersey and my Bears hat, which I had embroidered, "#73 Jordan's Voice Against Bullying." I also had on my old-school Chicago Bears coat. My girlfriend was going with me to give me a hand, and she knew someone at the stadium who would allow us to put my banner on the rails in the end zone area. That was impressive to hear—now more people could see Jordan's cause. So, we headed out, because the game started at noon, and we needed time to do things as well as put the banner up and get petitions signed. My girlfriend would take pictures of people signing the petition with their permission. It was cold outside, and people were enjoying their tailgate parties, so I tried to get as many signatures as I could outside before heading in. We headed to the entrance so we could line up to get in early to hang the banner up, eager to get in because of the cold; having been out there since 9:00 a.m. was a bigger factor, though. The doors opened to let in people with early entrance tickets, and they allowed us to get in as well. We made it up to the Budweiser section and took the stairs down to the front row section to hang the banner. Then I headed back up to the Budweiser section and prepared the petitions to be signed inside; we grabbed something to drink, and as we moved around, we told people about our cause, and people signed. I also was handing out the business cards for Jordan's site so people would have one on hand in case they forgot. From that point on, I was passing the petition up and down rows, explaining to people what it was for. I received hugs from ladies and some guys, along with a lot of handshakes, as people let me know they were sorry and that I was a strong person to be doing what I was doing.

As the game progressed, I turned and looked when the crowd roared loudly and began thinking what it would be like if Jordan were there with me watching the game. Tears filled my eyes, and I would have to wipe them. My throat was dry and would crack at times, so I would have to take a break and get a drink and return. It was hard repeating his story, as my heart was hurting, and numbness filled part of my body while chills filled the rest. I had to do this—no one else was going to—and even though I had people say, "I have your back," the only real backing was God keeping me together mentally and my girlfriend helping me as much as she could, giving me moral support. Besides that, no one was giving me assistance! I know people are sorry and say, "I will pray for you." I had friends in the county where my son lived who never came to his funeral to give me support because they were distancing themselves from me, fearing backlash from the community and politics. I already knew this from my prior dealing with state corrections; I knew how people turned on you, leaving you sitting all alone, wondering if you were going to make it or be a statistic. I was hoping people would take bullying to heart and rally around me, but I just figured they saw a stern-looking man who worked as a correctional officer so he could deal with the emotion. Yes and no! Jordan, like my other two children, I loved, but Jordan and I had that special father-and-son bond; we had a lot in common, and his emotional capacity was as mine was when I was his age. I was bullied while living in Cicero from kindergarten all the way to fifth grade. If I had not had that break until the harassment in corrections, I might not have made it either. God was preparing me for this moment when I asked him years ago to give me strength, perseverance, and hope to continue. Jordan just wanted to be friends with everyone and try and make people laugh when they were down; he was a great kid and the best son that any person could hope for.

I got back to getting the petitions signed. When the game was over, we headed out. The Bears lost the game, and we were both very tired. We drove back to my place, and my girlfriend gave me a hug, then left to get home and get ready for work the next day. I woke up the next morning for a new work week, still very tired from standing on my feet all day at the football game and telling Jordan's story repeatedly to the point my throat was sore and scratchy, and I could hardly talk. I made it out of bed and into the shower, got dressed, then headed out. I stopped by the local fast-food place and picked up some breakfast and headed to work. This seemed like the hardest part of the day as I continued forward. At times, I just wanted to grab the phone and call in and veg out in front of the television or the computer all day, not being bothered by anyone.

I arrived at work. The routine was the same. Not much was going on, and the day went by smoothly. That was great, because Tuesday, I had to head back down to my son's school with my attorney and his assistant for the school board meeting. I had researched online and learned that several children had taken their own lives due to bullying. The numbers may not seem very high, but when you look at it, one out of five children between middle school and high school report being bullied each year (National Center for Education Statistics). Plus, kids who are bullied are two to nine times more likely to commit suicide than children who have not been bullied. Further, 165,000 children a day skip school or pretend to be sick because they don't want to be confronted by their bullies, and 65 percent of all teen suicides are caused by bullying; and the bullying doesn't always happen at school. Sometimes it happens at home as well.

Tuesday arrived. The morning work routine came and went, and then I was off to my son's school. I had gassed up early that morning, so I stopped at a drive-through for a sandwich and a drink and headed down. My drive consisted of talking to God and asking for a positive result. I arrived and waited for my family to show. I did not see my attorney, and it was getting close to time for the meeting to begin. My mom and sister arrived. As we walked to the meeting room, there was my attorney and his assistant; they had entered through the front of the school. He looked around and said, "Where are the three police officers?" I was shocked. I said, "Probably someone told them I wasn't coming, because I did say I wasn't." So the superintendent felt safer thinking I was not going to be there; that showed they valued their lives more than those of the children in the school. I mentioned to my attorney that when I was at the first meeting, they were presenting a slideshow and revealed they received a $1.3 million antibullying grant from the federal government at the beginning of 2013, but there was nothing to show for it.

Jordan's Voice

The meeting began, and I signed my name to speak. The first part of the meeting was another slideshow about how well educated their children were compared to those in the rest of the state and how they had no problems with their program. Then the superintendent spoke and said that their police department would fill out the forms for a federal grant so they could have a police officer walking the halls. I raised my hand, interrupting, and said, "Why now and not a number of years back, like other schools in the Southern region? I heard the police wanted to do it before, but the school officials did not want a negative or threatening appearance around the children." The superintendent bounced back and replied, "Surely it wasn't me that said that."

They went on to talk about their anonymous tip line where a child could go online and report issues occurring at school using their PIN number so that only the office would know. One lady said, "When was this started?" The superintendent said, "It has been in place since 2009." The lady replied, "My daughter and son go to school here, and they are not aware of this, nor do they have a PIN number." She went on, "There is nothing in the student handbook mentioning any tip line; will it be in next year's handbook?" The superintendent said, "We have changed companies, and they do not have the PIN numbers changed over yet, but it will be done soon."

I looked at my attorney and shook my head as if to say, "Wow!" So, being me and wanting answers, I raised my hand and said, "Mr. Superintendent, can you tell me since March 2012, when the governor signed the Antibullying Bill HB5290, how many kids have been suspended for bullying?" The school board president stepped in and said those were things the superintendent would have to look up. I replied, "Here is an easier question: How many kids have been expelled from school since then for physical bullying or harassment?" The school board president again replied for the superintendent and said, "These are questions you need to put in writing, and we will come back to you with a timely response."

My attorney leaned over and said, "Good questions. What they're saying is, write your questions down, and they will give it to their attorneys and reply to you with what they want me to hear and not the truth."

There was another parent who complained that their child in kindergarten did not want to ride the bus or go to school because there were a couple of first and second graders hitting on him and teasing him. The superintendent asked, "Have you said something to the teacher, and how have they managed it?" The parent said they were going to look into it. Then the superintendent said, "I will talk to the principal and teacher." Another parent mentioned that their daughters and son had been bullied and nothing had been done about it. We listened, and when the meeting was over, we headed out to the lunch commons area. My attorney spoke to one lady and was shocked by what she had been told by the principal and his actions toward her children. I talked just a bit with my attorney, and they said they would be calling me later with details, but that he could see they were dodging a bullet. I said goodbye to my mom and sister and to others and headed back home.

The drive was the same: thinking about the responses I had received and looking over at the passenger seat, remembering the drive back to my place when he was with me. A tear rolled down my face and then another, then the floodgates opened, and my chest began to hurt. I was not having a heart attack or anxiety; I was in deep loss without my little buddy with me, feeling how empty I was without him. Things were beginning to change inside me—how I viewed things and how I approached situations. I started slowly shutting people out a little at a time, trying to figure out how to approach each problem and solve it if I could so I could get to the other problems at hand as well. I made it home and took a quick shower; it felt great. Then I grabbed my meds and went to bed. I laid down, and in my mind, I thanked God for keeping me together and not letting me break down amid this.

I started having trouble with Beth, because she wanted me to recap everything in a post on Jordan's Facebook page. I had my girlfriend type everything I had to say so there would not be any grammatical errors. I posted it, and soon after, I got a reply from Beth: "Brad, did you write this, or did your girlfriend?" I replied, "I did it on WordPerfect, and it was my words." Beth replied. "I'm done; I told you I didn't want to be collaborating with your girlfriend, because I don't think she is very supportive, and she is not behind this." I then stated, "Beth, she isn't collaborating with you; she was helping me with grammatical errors." She then came out and stated, "I don't like being deceived, and I'm out." I said, "OK, then give me all the passcodes for the site, and I will try and run it myself."

I was floored. This lady was talking to my girlfriend, telling her to back away because I needed to let God heal me, and she was talking to my daughter, trying to counsel her and causing disruption. I sent her a text: "Please do not be talking to my daughter or my family, and you are no longer part of this project." I really didn't know what to think at this time. This lady had come into my life saying that the Holy Spirit had spoken to her, telling her to assist me so Jordan's death would not be in vain, and I believed her and then was dropped because I wouldn't run my son's site in the way she wanted. She wanted my complete attention all the time; after I got off work, there was either a voicemail or text messages saying, "Contact me as soon as possible."

My girlfriend said, "I can't believe how much this woman's behavior has changed, back and forth." I agreed! I called my attorney's office and told his assistant about the situation, informing her that Beth was not part of Jordan's Voice and there was no reason for her to contact them except to give them the log-on information and passwords. I started saying to myself that I wished when people said something, they stood behind it or supported you. I noticed when Beth posted on the website, there weren't a lot of views, but when I posted things, I would receive twenty to forty thousand views (compared to three to four thousand on her posts). Sometimes things she would post were her opinions and based on an open standard, offending certain religious beliefs or sexual beliefs. I did not want a site criticizing people or judging people; I wanted everyone who opposed bullying to come together and voice their opinions about how they felt bullying had affected them or their children. My attorney's assistant said, "We will deal with this."

The rest of November consisted of a daily ritual, as did the first part of December; I would get off from work and go to the surrounding towns and walk the shopping areas and businesses and ask people to sign the petition, spending a couple of hours a day doing that. I had the approval of a local bowling alley to come every night during league gatherings and have people sign. I found that by the evening's end, my voice was all scratchy, and I would have to have something to drink and take a spoonful of honey when I got home. Sometimes someone would ask, "Was this your son?" and my throat would dry up, and I would softly say, "Yes, he was my little buddy." Some guys would shake my hand, and some women would give me a hug and say, "You are so strong doing what you are doing, trying to make a positive change."

    I did another interview with Channel 4 out of Saint Louis before the holidays. It consisted of me, a Missouri principal from one of the local towns, and a sci-fi guy who would use *Star Wars* characters to reach out to instruct kids about bullying. The principal spoke about how their anonymous tip line had decreased bullying in their school by 60 to 70 percent, which was a large decrease. At Jordan's school, they said they had one, but nothing about it was stated in their student handbook, and some parents said their children never received a PIN number. I had a chance to speak at the beginning of the segment and quickly at the end. The thing was, there was not a whole lot of time to really reflect on how bullying is overlooked and ignored. I answered the questions with short responses, because time was limited, but inside, I wanted to explode with what parents and children had told me; I wanted to talk about how I was bullied and how it affected me in life. There are outcomes to bullying, and 80 percent of them are bad. The only thing is that our society is willing to accept the death, or suicide, ratio because it is lower than the survival ratio. I am a survivor of bullying, whether it was physical, verbal, mental, or political; I have survived perhaps because I am stubborn enough to say I do not care what someone else thinks or because I was afraid of what I might do, and the fear of God kept me from doing something that I would have regretted. I will stand up for my rights, and if I am not wrong, you better believe I will strongly stand up, and I will stand up for my son.

    Since all this happened, I had to put together a way to raise money to pay for the rest of the funeral cost and headstone. I ended up taking the sniper rifle that I bought to give him when he went into the military, and I started a raffle. My mother and sister sold about thirty tickets, then between

Jordan's Voice

a gun armory shop, and I went to gun shows throughout the southern part of the state, where they let me set up a table to raffle off the gun. The gun cost me $3,000; I was able to raise $15,000 and pay for everything and put my dad's information on the back side of the headstone—all there had been for him before was a ground plaque from Veterans Affairs, because my stepmother couldn't afford a headstone. I also had ceramic pictures of my dad and Jordan placed on the headstone so people could remember them at their best. Jordan was in his football uniform, and my dad's picture was of him when he was younger, in his military uniform. There were four gun shows I attended from 8:00 a.m. to 4:00 p.m. At each show, I had his banners up and pictures of him on the table; this was from January to March. The weekends at the gun show were long, and my voice would get weak from telling people about the raffle and what it was for. Some would ask how it happened. Several people had a feeling and asked, "Was he your son?" I would keep tears from falling, even though they filled my eyes, and then they would give me big hugs. These were hard moments, especially when I had the laptop computer continuously playing his memorial video, and the last song that would play was "He's, My Son." That would always make a tear fall, goosebumps rise on my arms, and my stomach feel empty. Then when the show was over, I would thank Bob, who oversaw the gun shows, for letting me be there and Allen and his wife for sharing with me a table to display the rifle. These are people who really did not know me and reached out to allow me to do this and gave me assistance because I was doing it for a great cause. I never received any help from Jordan's mom or her family or friends; I didn't really care, because that showed me how selfish and self-centered some people can be. I know she is hurting, and she has a lot of pain inside, and she will carry what her part was in his death.

 I signed up for the state's 2014 Conference for Teen and Young Adult Suicide Prevention. It took place on April 25, 2014, and was held at the college in our state capital. It was a full day of seminars, training lectures, and guest speakers who covered the complete details of some programs. The main problem was the state having to find a way to integrate these programs into the educational curriculum, because children were expected to learn more at an earlier age. I am not saying this cannot be done, but it must be reinforced at an early age.

I went through some down moments in 2014, dealing with Jordan's death and dealing with issues of my own at work. I continued to campaign with his advocacy and get my paperwork done to go back to school. There were times I did not know if I was going to continue. Tad, my attorney, filed a lawsuit against the football coach, the principal of the school, the superintendent, the police department, and the company that showed the video. The company that showed the video explained they did not see how their video could be a triggering mechanism and that they had never had any issues before. When we researched the video they presented to the children on October 16, 2013, we found they had shown photos of children who had succeeded in committing suicide. In December 2013, the company stated on their website that the last portion of their video was replaced with a music video and the photos of kids were removed. This reflected the old saying, "If it is not broken, why fix it?" especially after the death of a child went national. The police department slid their way out of the lawsuit, citing a clause stating it is not their responsibility to make sure people get assistance if there is deemed to be no danger, but obviously, the officers who responded to the call did not have any suicide prevention or crisis intervention training. The call came in at 9:06 p.m. to dispatch; the officer arrived at his house, talked to him and his mother, and was gone by 9:16 p.m. Simply put, there was not enough time to gather enough information to determine if the child was in danger, even for the officer or his mother to look at his text messages to see what he had said to Alexis, whom he told what he was going to do.

During this period in 2014, I did go to the state capital with a proposal for stronger guidelines making it mandatory that children go to counseling for bullying. I went to every state representative and state senator to plead my case, and all they did was put together a House resolution to honor his memory and the fact that he died due to a cruel behavior called bullying, and every person should reflect on his death and how we treat other people. The resolution was signed December 3, 2014, before the changes in the House of Representatives in the state; this was just the start of me pushing a proposal for a bill.

The pictures below are of letters I sent at the end of January 2014 and a letter I received back from President Obama. I sent the letter out before the incident in Ferguson, Missouri, when a black man was shot by a police officer and then forty to sixty FBI agents were sent to go door-to-door to investigate the shooting. The conclusion from three separate investigations was the same: the shooting was justified because of his actions. Why do we not investigate incidents of suicide to the extent we do shootings that people feel are racial? The law describes everyone, no matter their race, creed, sexual orientation, or religion, as protected.

BRADLEY L. LEWIS

To: President Barack Obama

From: Mr. Bradley L. Lewis

Dear Mr. President

I'm sending you this letter in hopes that you would take this seriously and understand that our children of this nation are suffering from a behavior that has gone on way to long. The behavior I speak of is "Bullying" and it comes in many ways and forms and affects everyone from grade school children from K-12th grade, then carries over into college and then adult life. There are many statistics out there supporting the short and long term effects of what bullying does to a person.

Why is this important to me? My son Jordan Robert Lewis took his life the morning of October 17, 2013 after his mother and her boyfriend left for work. Jordan took the shot gun of his mother's boyfriend and shot himself in the heart after leaving a suicide letter stating "that bullying has caused him to do this and those of you know who you are."

Jordan was a wonderful boy, always wanting to be friends with anyone and would always try and make the girls laugh. He was very helpful and kind and would stand up for others, he was unselfish and had a soft heart and never knew a stranger like his grandpa Lewis. He never had a chance to grow up and contribute his love and kindness because bullying was too much for him and like others when you feel there is no out you take the quickest route to end the pain.

The school district does not want to acknowledge and says there were never any official documents that he was ever bullied on school grounds. When a child goes and tells a teacher or a football coach and even a principle that is not official unless they do their job and document it themselves.

I only found out about some bullying a month before he died and that is because he wasn't acting the same and was quiet. I finally was able to get him to tell me, but he said "You would not understand" I replied and said "You would be surprised what dad has been thru in life". He stated he was being bullied and picked on and I told him to go to the teacher or principle and let them know about it and then let me know. I told him not to worry about what the other kids think about you telling and to let me know what they say so I could follow up. During that month when I talk to him how school was going and how his grades were, he would reply everything is good and his grades are good as well.

Thursday morning around 7:30am I was at my post at South Western Illinois Correctional Center getting everything ready for when count cleared and I received the call from my ex-wife that my son is dead and that he shot himself. My heart stopped and my stomach dropped, my little buddy was dead..... There must be something wrong he wouldn't shoot himself!!!

The thing Mr. President is, there have been a lot of children take their lives over the years because of bullying and I know because I'm a survivor and it goes on even in the work place as kids get older and become adults, through sexual, gender, religious, social, political harassment. We take ethic test every year in our state, your state and the political and personnel biasness is there. There are so many violations of ethics, but they tend to cover them up with the gray areas of contracts and AD's and ID's and union articles.

I'm reaching out as an advocate for bullying and all individuals who have been affected or are being affected by this behavior. Bullying has a short immediate affect which is suicide, the longer terms are individuals being introverted and withdrawing from society and feel they have no purpose. The next affect is a person becomes stronger and deals with life head on and is a survivor, but the last affect is the victim becomes the bully and either they continue the heartless behavior or they become the people in prison who decided to take matters in their own hands and the outcome is horrific with school shootings and other situations like the movie theater shooting out west.

Bradley L. Lewis

I'm trying to push on my son's web site Jordan's Voice Against Bullying a federal petition for Anti Bullying law that would mandate all schools in the United States who receive federal money to be held accountable to document all complaints of bullying by parents or children that is brought forward. I have also attached a copy of the petition in the envelope to share what are some ideas and that there are even more I would like to share. I will also be sending same letters to other U.S. representatives as well as my attorney who is dealing with my son's case so everything is documented for this petition and that no one can say they never received any official documentation.

Thank You Very Much Mr. President

Sincerely: Bradley L. Lewis

P.S. Please help the children and the families of this country feel their child's death was not in vain.

THE WHITE HOUSE
WASHINGTON

August 6, 2014

Mr. Bradley L. Lewis
Collinsville, Illinois

Dear Bradley:

　　Thank you for writing. I am deeply saddened to learn of the loss of your son, Jordan, and the pain you have experienced.

　　Words fail when a loved one is taken from us too soon, and as a parent my heart breaks for the young lives lost to bullying. Bullying in all its forms is unacceptable, and I am committed to ensuring our schools and communities are places where all Americans can feel safe to learn, grow, and work toward achieving their dreams.

　　Please know I will keep all those affected by bullying in my thoughts and prayers.

Sincerely,

[signature: Barack Obama]

I have talked to parents on my son's Facebook site and heard more stories of kids being bullied severely and others taking their lives. In June 2014, just over a week after school ended at my son's school, a young girl of sixteen, someone he knew, committed suicide, shooting herself with her father's service revolver. Even though the papers did not say much about it, the whispers of bullying spread; she was a girl who responded on Jordan's Facebook site and would talk about herself being bullied because she was gay.

The pictures you see below are crime scene photos from Jordan's suicide. Please understand I am showing these photos to allow people to see how far a child will go to try to end the pain and suffering if nothing can be done to protect them.

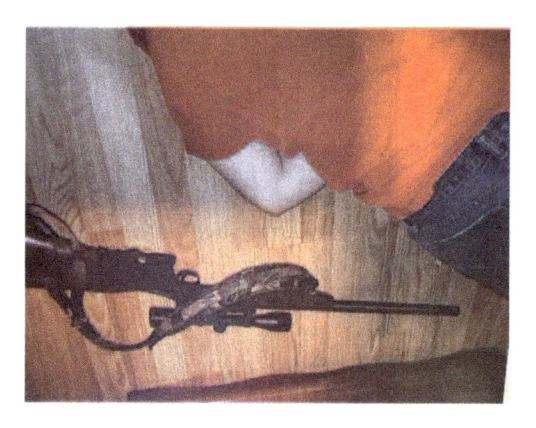

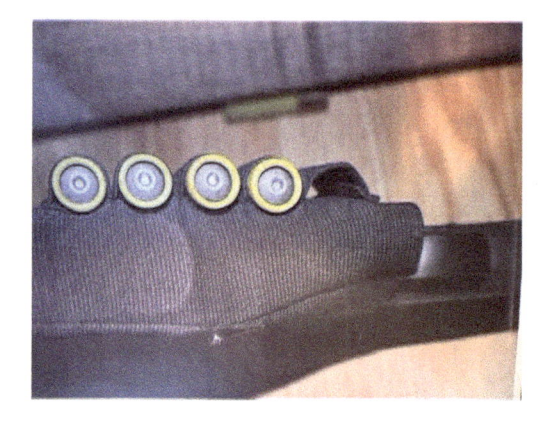

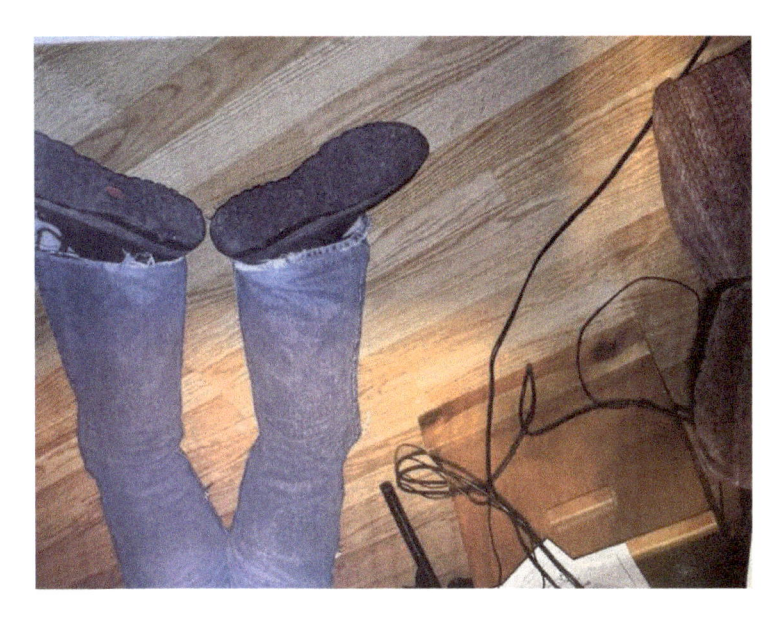

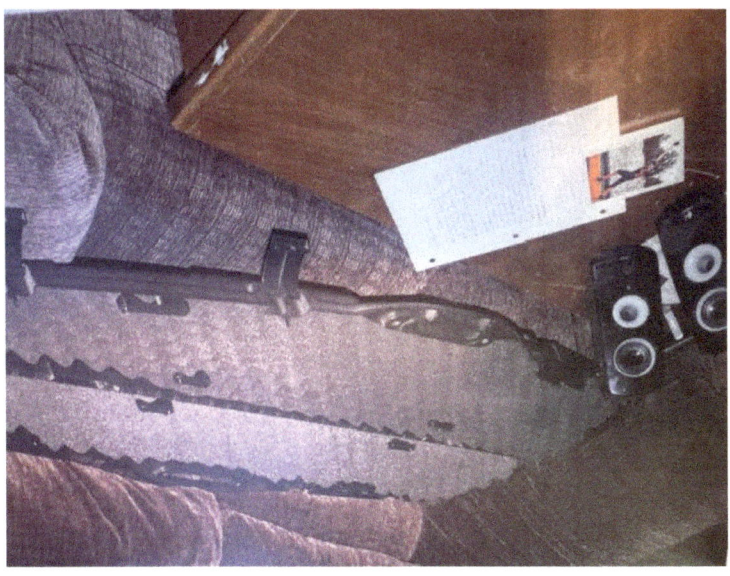

These are crime scene photos of Jordan's death; others are not available due to being too graphic for publication and too horrific for the public to view.

CHAPTER ELEVEN

This is the proposal I wrote for our state and sent to my federal representative so that it would be considered to help kids and force schools to properly document all forms of bullying. If it takes placing teeth in a bill, so be it.

★ ★ ★

6/23/2014

Dear Honorable Sir/Madam,

Subject: Proposal for (Jordan's Voice Against Bullying), a bill which would be made into law.

Definition: Bullying.

Bullying is unwanted, aggressive behavior among school-aged children that involves a real or perceived power imbalance. The behavior is repeated, or has the potential to be repeated, over time. Both kids who are bullied and kids who bully others may have serious, lasting problems.

In order to be considered bullying, the behavior must be aggressive and include:

- An Imbalance of Power: Kids who bully use their power—such as physical strength, access to embarrassing information, or popularity—to control or harm others. Power imbalances can change over time and in different situations, even if they involve the same people.

- Repetition: Bullying behaviors happen more than once or have the potential to happen more than once.

Bullying includes actions such as making threats, spreading rumors, attacking someone physically or verbally, and excluding someone from a group on purpose.

- Types of Bullying
- Where and When Bullying Happens
- Frequency of Bullying

Types of Bullying

There are three types of bullying:

- Verbal bullying is saying or writing mean things. Verbal bullying includes:
  - Teasing
  - Name-calling
  - Inappropriate sexual comments
  - Taunting
  - Threatening to cause harm

- Social bullying, sometimes referred to as relational bullying, involves hurting someone's reputation or relationships. Social bullying includes:
  - Leaving someone out on purpose
  - Telling other children not to be friends with someone
  - Spreading rumors about someone
  - Embarrassing someone in public

- Physical bullying involves hurting a person's body or possessions. Physical bullying includes:
  - Hitting/kicking/pinching
  - Spitting
  - Tripping/pushing
  - Taking or breaking someone's things
  - Making mean or rude hand gestures

We propose a bill that would mandate that all schools in the United States, whether they receive federal money or not … follow the guidelines and policies that are enacted in the following proposals and would criminalize the act of bullying in all public educational institutions nationwide—a federal bill.

We seek in this bill *zero tolerance* between school administration, teachers, school board members, professors, deans, district bus drivers, parent volunteers, counselors and minors in their care, and peer to peer.

We seek in this bill that any student/athlete found to be bullied, whether it be verbally or physically … be mandated to counseling. And in the event the student continues to bully during or after the conclusion of counseling, the student/athlete bullying may be subject to disciplinary action by state and/or federal laws—whichever law has the broader reach—to ensure that the student/athlete bullying be encouraged to cease and desist from continuing in such injurious behavior.

We further request that under such guidelines listed above, listed under verbal or social bullying, any student/athlete found to be verbally bullying by means of personal contact, phone, electronic devices, letters, offensive pictures, gestures, excluding individuals from partaking in any groups or social events, or even having others doing their bidding that this student/athlete is mandated to counseling and that the following discipline be considered.

First Offense: A student/athlete will be suspended for one to three days of school. The suspension will involve community service in the district or with the special education department, assisting teachers or teachers' assistants in helping the special needs children during the school day.

Furthermore, the student/athlete will be required to attend one hour of counseling sessions with a licensed counselor, and a parent/guardian will be present, but not involved, in the session.

Unless required by the counselor, before the student/athlete can return to school, the session must be signed off on by the counselor and documented through the school's district office. All counseling fees will be paid by the student/athlete's parents, and no fees will be incurred by the school district for the counseling. All schoolwork will be completed and turned in with credit, and quizzes/tests/exams will be made up on the student's free time after regular school hours if the student/athlete adheres to the guidelines.

Second Offense: A student/athlete will be suspended for three to five days of school, and the suspension will involve the same as the first offense, whereas the counseling session will increase to two separate one-hour sessions, and the parent/guardian will be required to attend counseling by a licensed counselor but will not be involved unless directed by the counselor. Furthermore, the student's/athlete's parents will be responsible for all costs during the counseling sessions as part of their responsibility so that no cost will be incurred by the school district. Furthermore, if the student/athlete or parent/guardian refuses to attend the counseling session, the student/athlete will not be allowed to return to school unless the session is documented and confirmed by the counselor and documentation is received by the school district. All assignments will be completed and credited as that of quizzes/test/exams that may be made up on student's time after regular school hours if the student/athlete adheres to the guidelines.

Third Offense: If a student's/athlete's bullying behavior continues, expulsion from the current school will take place, and if applicable, they will be recommended to an alternative school that deals strictly with children with behavioral issues as their own, not placing them with children with more severe issues but making sure that the student/athlete be given the ability to develop the proper social skills to succeed in society.

We further request under such guidelines that any student/athlete found to be in violation of the school's bullying guidelines and who harms another student/athlete by means of physical assault, which includes spitting, hitting, kicking, pinching, tripping, throwing items at another, breaking another student's/athlete's property, or instigating another student/athlete to do the same to another student/athlete will be disciplined as follows.

First Offense: A student's/athlete's parents will be called to the school; local law enforcement will be notified as well. Depending on the nature of the offense and the severity, if the victim's parents/guardians agree not to press any charges, the student/athlete before returning to school will be given a one-week suspension and will have to agree along with their parents/guardians that they undergo a period of counseling and anger management sessions and that the parents/guardians must attend but not be involved, provided that the licensed counselor or physician does not require their involvement. If the student/athlete or parent/guardian refuses to comply with attendance or guidelines required, the student/athlete will be expelled from the current school, and if local law enforcement deems, charges may be enforced by the state's attorney in the district. Furthermore, if the student/athlete and their parents/guardians agree, and all guidelines are met, all assignments and homework can be completed during the student's/athlete's suspension along with quizzes/test/exams so no lapse in education occurs.

Second Offense: Parents/guardians will be called in, local law enforcement will be notified, and the student/athlete will be expelled from school. The student/athlete will be subject to state and local laws for bullying, assault, and any other violations that occur due to the incident.

We further request in the event bullying makes/drives/forces an individual to take their own life/commit suicide/end their life prematurely that the responsible party or parties be charged under special state and/or federal law(s) which shall designate bullying as a violent hate crime.

We further request in the event bullying makes/drives/forces an individual to take their own life/commit suicide/end their life prematurely that the responsible party or parties be charged for no lesser a charge than that of involuntary manslaughter, and where the perpetrator(s) are found to have encouraged or egged on the individual by daring or recommending that the individual take their own life, the charges be elevated to manslaughter.

We also seek in this bill that all school administrators, teachers, school board members, professors, deans, coaches, parent volunteers, and counselors in the school systems (whether volunteer or stipend) go through mandatory preventative training, crisis intervention training, suicide prevention training, and up-to-date training in the ways students go about creating new ways to bully and harass other students; that such training is no less than two full days of classroom training, group workshops, and seminars by specialists in these fields before the school year begins; that documentation shall be on file and available when requested when an incident occurs; and that certified proof shall be readily available showing up-to-date training has been done.

We also seek in this bill that complete guidelines be taught to the students and written out in detail on school websites and in handbooks to be given to parents who are not computer savvy or who cannot afford a computer or internet that completely spell out, so there is no misunderstanding, what bullying is or that a person decides to report bullying when there is no bullying occurring. If bullying does occur, it will be documented so that patterns can be shown of the abuse from the person bullying or the victim being bullied.

We also seek in this bill that school administrators, teachers, school board members, professors, deans, coaches, district bus drivers, parent volunteers, and counselors in the school systems (whether volunteer or stipend) also be held accountable if he/she/they ignore, brush off, or discourage students from reporting acts of bullying on themselves or witnessing acts of bullying against others in any manner (i.e., intimidation, ridicule, and/or disregarding the emotional impact the bullying is having on the student reporting the bullying incident[s]).

We also seek in this bill that school administrators, teachers, school board members, professors, deans, coaches, district bus drivers, parent volunteers, and counselors in the school systems (whether volunteer or stipend) also be held accountable if he/she/they engage in or fail to appropriately make a record of and remedy any incidents of reported bullying made to them by students/parents occurring within an educational day, whether it be before, during, or after school, to include any off-campus extracurricular activities such as field trips, sporting events, or bus transportation to and from campus. Failure to abide by these guidelines would result in punishment by state and federal laws and fines and imprisonment if injuries occur to a child as a result of lack of professionalism and job responsibilities.

We also seek in this bill that if schools ignore the policies put in place and refuse to document any reports of bullying because it could affect their image, the image of the community, the image of candidates in office, or the image of a prestigious family in the community, the school will have their accreditation reviewed and points could be removed, lowering their accreditation grade and impacting their overall federal funding.

We also seek in this bill that schools allow for the presence of a uniformed officer during school hours and that all reported incidents of bullying be documented by the school administrators, teachers, school board members, professors, deans, coaches, parent volunteers, and counselors in the school systems (whether volunteer or stipend) receiving the report and be provided to local law enforcement and that all electronic devices reported to be used in the act of bullying be immediately taken into possession and handed over to law enforcement for investigation.

We also seek in this bill that law enforcement have the right to interview any minor student(s)/athlete(s) who knowingly witness an act or acts of bullying against another minor as part of a thorough investigation with a lawyer/parent/guardian present during the interview in an effort to remedy the bullying and save the victim and other potential victims from the threat of physical or mental harm and/or loss of life as a cause or result of the effects of bullying.

In the event of a suicide or death known or alleged to be the result of acts of bullying, law enforcement will immediately seize possession of all social networking accounts, cell phones, laptops, and any other form of electronic device that may have been used in acts of bullying against the deceased victim as well as the victim's electronic devices and accounts in order to conduct a complete and thorough investigation.

We also seek in this bill that better educational programs be created and implemented into the general educational base from preschool through high school so that social and behavioral skills can be developed properly at a younger age and hopefully be reinforced each year in all school activities; the students can use these skills to better their lives and careers so no child feels left out or feels that the world would be a better place without them, because every child's life makes a difference in this world.

We also seek in this bill that the United States Department of Education make anti-bullying education a priority in the nationwide curriculum, including the appropriate allocation of funding in an amendment to the president's 2015 budget proposal for education and that the funding percentage allocated be no less than that funding currently allocated to implement the development and execution of other educational programs and agendas geared toward protection, equality, and health of students such as D.A.R.E. and other school safety/security programs, as noted in the president's 2014 budget proposal for education, which stated:

[For] each state that involves themselves in the collection of lotteries, casino gambling, and video gambling machines in establishments ... proceeds will be used for all school educational programs. [Money] which is allocated to the state education budget by the state legislation will not be redirected for other uses and replaced with gambling proceeds collected from state gambling earnings. The money which is received from the federal government for education is directed directly to the state board of education school budget and not used for any other means.

We also seek in this bill that consequences for violating these guidelines be enforced and that federal fines be issued to school districts, to state boards of education, or to any public service network which includes police departments (city, county, and state), state social service offices, state attorney's offices, or public officials (city, county, state, and federal) who fail to comply with these guidelines or try to interfere or cover up any incidents of bullying to secure their community from any public embarrassments; they will be held accountable to the fullest. Fines will be directed to an account created to assist individuals who are recovering from the distress of bullying and outside group programs to assist students outside of school.

"...the president's plan to increase school safety and to decrease gun violence includes investments not only to prepare schools for emergencies, but also to create nurturing school climates and help children recover from the effects of living in communities plagued by persistent violence and abuse.

We also request that any petition signatures, waiving duplicates, from petitions that include the name(s) "Jordan's Law," "Make a Law for Jordan," Jordan Robert Lewis, "Jordan's Voice Against Bullying," "Jordan's Voice," or any other anti-bullying petition formed for Jordan Robert Lewis shall be included and counted in this petition.

In conclusion: A child grows and is nurtured by their surroundings. If a child is taught bullying at home or is not shown right from wrong, then the behavior goes undetected or is completely ignored, allowing them to behave any way they like.

The heart is a muscle in the body that pumps blood, which is our life support to every organ in our body, which allows us to survive. Over time, if we do not take care of our bodies, the heart grows weak, and our bodies will then shut down and die. The heart is the strongest muscle in the human body, but it also can become the weakest. The heart can be broken like the spirit of a wild horse once running free and wild. There are times when things happen to us through relationships, deaths, or others who are heartless and have no compassion for another's feelings. Over the span of our existence, the fabric of our societies has been torn apart by what we have allowed to happen because of our lack of seeing outside the box and learning from our past mistakes in life. Our society is in such a decline, and we the people are to blame for not stepping up and having the courage to demand a positive change so that our future relies on the proper development of teaching our children how to get along with one another and show respect before respect is given. The society of this world has manipulated and brainwashed children's minds to become heartless and cruel beings to learn to fight and to be their future weapons of tomorrow. Our future is set upon our children's ability to learn behavior, so let us make sure that we teach them love and compassion and that your actions affect the lives of others around you. To lose a life so precious as the life of Jordan Robert Lewis, who had so much love and kindness to share with everyone around him, is to have denied this world of something so

wonderful that only the memories of the ones who were able to know him can share his love through themselves.
 Sincerely,
 Bradley L. Lewis (the voice of Jordan Robert Lewis)

CHAPTER TWELVE

In October 2014, just shy of a year after Jordan's death, there was a twelve-year-old boy from the town my son had lived in that ended up shooting himself, but nothing much was really said. The story was that his mother died, and he was depressed, then the story from the paper was that it was an accidental shooting, and he was shot accidentally while cleaning his hunting rifle. Now, it's amazing that three kids in one year shot themselves in the same town. You could say it's a coincidence, but there have been parents who pulled their kids out of the district to homeschool them to keep them away from being bullied. Parents stated they complained, but the school ignored the complaints, and some families were afraid of retaliation and backed down. A parent should not have to be afraid to report that their child is being harmed or in danger of being harmed physically or mentally.

I have been through my own harassment at my job, before Jordan was born and before he died. In 2013, I interviewed for sergeant positions and didn't receive them, even though I was a senior person. I was refused inside training, which is six points on an interview. I placed twenty-five requests between 2013 and 2016 and was refused on everyone except one that was approved by the warden, but he knew they were discontinuing that training, so it was canceled. Then, in late 2014, I approached the warden about the training in his office and stated, "I'm coming to you like a man asking to go to training, because I'm automatically six points short going into an interview without that training." The warden then stated, "I'm glad you're coming to me like a man, but I wish you had done so before filing a grievance on me for refusing training; I might have been able to manipulate overtime to get you training." Wow! The first thing that entered my mind was, "You're retaliating against me for filing a justifiable grievance for violating a union contract?" I went home and wrote it up, and I went to our union president; his suggestion to me was, "Do not write him up, because it won't go right for you." I let it go, but I still kept the write-up. Then I went to the training lieutenant for copies of all my requests, and his reply was, "Lewis, there is no reason to ask them for your interview; they're not going to give you points or the training. Do you want to get promoted?" I said, "Yes!" The lieutenant said, "You're going to have to exploit your son's death, because they're not going to promote you any other way than that." I was shocked! "So that is how it is done and how I will get promoted?" I asked. The lieutenant replied, "Yes."

I left the training office and went to our union vice president. I told him, then told the shift commander. The next day, I was talking to our other shift commander and explained everything to him. He responded, "What a fucking idiot! Write it up and give me the original after you make yourself a copy." The incident happened on a Wednesday, and I wrote the report on that Thursday. On Friday, the warden approached me in the employee dietary and nudged me on the elbow, then said, "I heard what happened, and we will take care of it." I replied to the warden, "I expect you to deal with it, because it was totally unprofessional and unethical, and I will also pursue this myself, letting my attorney know."

I went home that evening, aggravated over the whole thing, thinking how morbid this guy was for suggesting I do that. I was off from work that Saturday and Sunday and came back to work on Monday. I was assigned to my zone in the shack, watching all housing movement. Well, that lieutenant I wrote up was assigned to my zone. In the first part of the morning, he would walk from the administration door to the housing units, looking my way and grinning at me. Then an hour later, he walked past the movement shack, looking in and smiling at me as he passed by. I was relieved for lunch a half hour later, and as I walked to the administration door and walked in, that lieutenant was walking across into the segregation and stopped and said to me while he was smiling, "Lewis, do you have a problem?" I continued walking on by and headed to the warden's office. When I approached the office, his secretary called the assistant warden and notified him I was outside his office; he called me in, and when I told him about the situation, he replied, "I will say something to the warden about it; this is harassment."

I returned to my assignment at the movement shack and monitored the line movements. At approximately 11:45 a.m., the same lieutenant walked up to my movement shack and stuck his face against the screen. He stated, "Lewis, what's the problem? Come out." I replied, "Get away from the shack. You're not supposed to be speaking to me since I wrote you up." The lieutenant persisted and tried opening the door, but I had it locked. The lieutenant continued to try opening the door, telling me to open it. Then he stated, "Lewis, come out here and do your job." I replied, "I'm not coming out there with you." I then got on the phone and called the warden's office and told the warden, "Get this lieutenant away from my door; he is trying to force his way into the shack." The warden said he was notifying the shift commander and would have him send someone out to relieve me.

The entire time, I was on the phone with the warden, and even when the shift commander called me back and asked me to come to his office, the lieutenant was still telling me to open the door and saying, "What's the problem?" and "Why can't you come out and talk to me?" The lieutenant finally left, and another officer came out to relieve me so I could go to the warden's office. When I arrived at the warden's office, the shift commander and assistant warden of programs were there. I shut the door, and the warden asked me for the second time that day what was going on. I had to go through the whole thing for the third time that day, in addition to writing up the lieutenant two more times in one day, even after explaining the situation and stating that if they didn't do anything, I would file for an order of protection. I had a sergeant interview the following week, and I stated, "This is going to be held against me in my interview." They replied, "No, it won't." They had me go into another office so they could speak to the lieutenant. I couldn't hear anything, but when he left, they came in and told me they were going to look into it. I waited over two weeks and never heard a thing, then one morning when I was coming into work, our internal affairs lieutenant told me that there was not too much they could do because it was a "he said, she said" situation, and he had bigger fish to worry about. I was angry that nothing was going to be done and that they were going to overlook me again on the sergeant promotion because of the write-ups I submitted.

I went home that evening and wrote a letter to the department of corrections director, and had it notarized and sent it as certified mail so I could make sure they received it, then I made copies of the notarized letter and all documents I sent him. I was tired of being shat on and held back because I wasn't in the right political clique, or I didn't agree with things when they were managed the wrong way. The warden had told me in the past when I confronted him about training that he sent people to training who he thought were motivated. This was after he went to my son's funeral and knew I was running an advocacy group against bullying and doing FEMA, IEMA, and Department of Homeland Security training on the side, even after I registered for the spring semester in college to continue and finish my degree. I had 180 college credit hours, served fifteen years in the active and reserve army and the National Guard, had thirteen certificates from outside state and federal training, and had twenty-two years of service in the department, so where was I not motivated? How do you think I felt after this?

I never received a response from the director or anyone else, and this showed me I did not matter. I fell into what you could call a funk; others would call it a depression, and it got to the point where I would sit around and veg out front of the television and watch movies and really do nothing but go to work. My girlfriend would wonder why I didn't call and tell me that she had not seen me in weeks. I really didn't want to be around anyone. When I went to work, it was hard to look at the warden and administrators without feeling sick about being around them. They all knew what I was going through, and they knew I was doing a lot of state and federal training outside of state corrections to earn points for my promotion and advocating talking to parents whose children were enduring bullying in their schools. I felt more like a failure because I couldn't defend myself or my son or help other kids with their problems. I would sit back at night crying, alone, asking God, "Why did you allow Satan to take him away when I would have gladly taken his place?" I felt pain deep inside, like someone had shoved their hand inside me and was trying to pull what life I had out of me but then letting go after I had received enough pain to regain my composure. Then I would lay there in tears, my eyes exhausted from the crying, with the images of Jordan lying there in a pool of his own blood, dead, and then I would fall asleep.

I started getting on Jordan's Facebook page just once a month, spending a few hundred dollars to reach out to children and parents, and in December, after figuring out where I was going to take my classes for my degree, I finally finished getting my paperwork in order. I had to put a bump in to a three-to-eleven shift so I could take day classes, and I needed to put in my days-off bump as well. We were having people retiring and others getting ready to retire in January 2015, and two sergeant spots were coming open. As I mentioned, I had received thirteen official certificates in outside training besides my school classes, I had 180 college credit hours (equivalent to a master's degree), and the only reason I didn't have my degree was I couldn't figure math out. I had so many articles to read and assignments to finish and then had to prepare myself mentally for the sergeant interview; my days were busy. Then I was receiving requests for motions of discovery from my attorney that he had received from the defendant's attorneys.

I won't say much about the sergeant interview this time; they already knew who they were picking and who they didn't want to promote, so it would be a waste of breath trying to say too much about it. The interview came on Wednesday at nine. I was in cycle training, and that was a joke, because all they did in cycle training was throw a movie in and have you sign paperwork that you were trained. I went up front to the reception desk and waited till it was my turn for the interview, then the administrative assistant came out and called me to come back with him. I walked back to the warden's conference room, knocked on the door, and waited till they said, "Come in." I proceeded in and greeted the assistant warden, the major, and the administrative assistant. I gave each of them a copy of my résumé and all my education documents, certificates, and training documents, and then I sat down. They said, "We have all your other information already down, so we're just going to ask you about scenarios, and you give your response. Then we will read you an incident, and you write down the information and then write the report."

I gave my responses for the scenarios, but the incident report was different; they usually give you the incident on paper, and you go into the next room for ten minutes and write the report. This time, they read it really quickly, and you couldn't get all the information down properly; they had never done it this way before. I felt I had done really well on the questions and was not nervous at all. When I was finished, they asked if I had any further questions, then I turned and left the room.

I don't think it really mattered how I did—they manipulated my scores so much that it put me out of range, like they had in the last interview. The thing is, if you're the senior person going into the interview, you have to beat me by ten points, and all they have to do is fudge numbers on the parts they can manipulate, especially the verbal interview. I remember in one interview, they didn't give me points for education, saying I didn't show proof of my high school diploma. Well, you had to have a GED or high school diploma just to work there, and how could I have gone to college without a diploma? I was glad it was over so I could focus more on my midterm exams at school. I felt the longer I stayed in corrections, the dumber they would make me feel; no matter how much education I received or how hard I tried, they still wouldn't promote me to save their special sergeants on day shift, with their shift and their days off, because if I did get promoted, I would be senior because of my seniority.

The following Monday, March 9, 2015, I went to the state capital for appointments I had made with state legislators to speak with them about the bullying proposal I had written to strengthen the state laws already put into effect by implementing penalties against schools or their faculty for not documenting bullying complaints brought forth by children or their parents. I even spoke with one of the governor's senior advisers about the problems throughout the state, and even in our jobs. Since I started in corrections at the maximum facility years back, there had been a number of staff who had committed suicide; some may say there were outside issues, but there were a lot of on-the-job harassment issues as well. I found that this senior adviser had a brother who worked down there, and he had committed suicide as well. I told him I was sorry to hear that, because I knew firsthand all the bullying and harassment I had received from my peers and management. I wasn't the type to go out and party, because I had children and school I had to tend to. The fifteen years and eleven months I spent at that facility included some of the worst moments of my life, until I transferred to where I was now. I then told him of the issues I was dealing with at my facility with them fudging the interviews to keep from promoting me, because people talk to one another between facilities, especially if they worked with each other at some point.

I had meetings with several state representatives that day. I showed them the proposal and the crime scene photos of Jordan's death, along with the suicide letter he left. There were several of them in tears as I explained that somewhere else in the state, a fifteen-year-old girl hung herself at the school bus stop before the other kids arrived and left a suicide note at home for her mother. She stated in her note, "Bullying has caused me to do this!" How many stories have I heard from parents whose children have committed suicide, attempted and failed, or contemplated the thought of taking their lives? I remember hearing from someone close to Jordan and his mother that he tried prior to this by taking a bottle of Tylenol, and his mom knew about it. A few of the state representatives said they stood behind it 100 percent.

I was tired and ready to head home. I had a large blister on the back of my left foot that had busted and bled into my sock. My back was sore from walking back and forth between the capital building where some offices were, then going under the tunnel to where the other offices were in another building. While I was driving home, I looked up at the angel hanging from my rearview mirror; it had Jordan's name on it, and it looked like him. The tears ran down my cheeks, and my face felt like it was being pulled downward, like gravity was ten times stronger, and I couldn't even attempt to open my mouth. My mind was so much on him and wishing he were there with me. I was wishing I could have done something or had known the police were at his house the night before, because I would have come straight there and tried figuring something out. Why did he not say something to me when I texted him about the game I had bought him that night before he died? When I turned my head and looked at the passenger seat, I could see him singing "Hey Jude" by the Beatles. He would always tell me not to sing when that song played, because he wanted to sing it by himself. He was really good at remembering lyrics to songs and singing; he loved to sing in the vehicle, in the shower, and when we went to concerts, where he would enjoy himself.

I continued to drive home with memories and pain, just wanting to go home and take a hot shower. Then I doctored my blister, took my meds, and went to bed. I prayed to God, thanking him for being there, helping me get through the last few days, giving me strength to speak to the legislators, and for me not falling apart, and as I lay there with tears in my eyes after saying my prayer, I fell asleep.

The next morning, I woke about eight o'clock and lay there for a bit before getting up to do my laundry for the week and to study for my midterm, which had been canceled because of the bad weather the week before. I then took some time out and did a video on Facebook to let parents in my state know about the talks I had had with legislators and what they had said. I posted it and advertised it, spending two hundred dollars on the advertising.

On March 26, 2015, we finally received our grades from our sergeant interviews. They had already announced a week prior who received the two spots; as expected, it was two people with less seniority than the sergeants on day shift they were protecting. The grades were screwed up again: they gave me 49.666 points. On education, I went from 7 points to 5 points, and I went lower on incident report writing and still had no inside training points. On March 27, 2015, I called work, and an officer who also interviewed stated, "The union steward is filing a grievance for four of us who have been denied training and denied points for training and had points taken away for education." That afternoon, I went to work and asked the administrative office for copies of all my past interviews.

Later, during my lunch break, I noticed the warden was still at the facility, so I knocked on his door and requested to speak with him. The warden said, "Yes, come in." I came straight out with it and said, "I thought you said you were going to send me to training, and there are two people who have fourteen fewer years than me going to screeners training who were interviewing with me, then they screwed the scoring up again, taking away points from education and experience." The warden right away stated, "No, they didn't. I looked it over and verified." I stated, "How did I go from seven points on education down to five points this time?" He said, "You went to SIUC back in the nineties; they did classes in quarter hours." I stated, "All my classes are in semester hours. If you look at the transcripts, they will show quarter hours and semester hours, and I was in classes six straight years." I added, "There seems to be something wrong, because no matter what I do, the scoring of the points changes every time." Then the warden said, "You act like I have a conspiracy against you, and I have seen the things you stated I have said, and I don't appreciate you saying things I didn't say or putting words into my mouth." I then stated, "I didn't have to put words into your mouth, and everything I wrote in the incident reports was true, because I keep notes of everything, so there is no reason for me to lie. You can give me a lie detector test and see the truth." The warden was getting aggravated and so frustrated that he said the same thing back: "You can give me one too." I then said again, "I have nothing to lie about, and do you think I would jeopardize everything I have been working for and going to school for to lie about you and others abusing your authority and screwing with people's lives?" He looked at me with a look suggesting he didn't know what to say. Then I reminded him again that I was keeping all records of interviews and write-ups and there would be a time the truth would come out. He didn't like it, and even so, he had had someone in the past two interviews who was not management but a lapdog, and this person received a lieutenant spot on the next lieutenant interview. How does that work?

It got to the point where I contacted an associate director and asked about some things related to the interview points, and he asked, "Did you do an internship in college?" I replied, "Yes, I did four hundred and fifty hours as an acting casework supervisor at the juvenile facility." I then contacted our union president at the time and told him what the associate director said, and he replied, "I don't care what he says; the union will determine what is accepted or not, and I might not even send your grievance to third level." This was coming from a guy who had just made sergeant in the last interview, and if I were to make sergeant, it would put him on the back shift.

Things were winding down. I had finished finals, and I was getting close to my deposition for Jordan's case. I was keeping myself busy, riding twenty-five to thirty-five miles a day, up to sixty or seventy on Saturdays, or absorbing myself in movies at the theater. I did end up breaking up with my girlfriend, based on the fact it wasn't fair for her with all my drama and my not being very sociable, as well dealing with work crap and Jordan's lawsuit.

The deposition finally arrived, and we met with attorneys for the school district and an attorney representing the gentleman who put together the movie. The deposition took about four and a half hours in total, with three bathroom breaks and a chance to refill our cups of water. The attorney representing the school went first, asking about the order of protection that Jordan's mom had filed when he was three years old. I replied, "Two weeks after she filed it, the judge deemed it had no validity to it." That was exhibit number one, to make me look bad and unstable. The next questions were about whether Jordan had doctors. At the time we were married, his doctor was the one that delivered him, and he had a different one when living with his mother. Then they asked if he was taking any medicine for depression or anxiety and if he was seeing a psychiatrist, psychologist, or counselor. I told them, "No!" I never knew of him going to any doctor like that, and he was never on any type of medicine unless he had a cold or flu. Then the attorney for the school district began asking me questions about comments that were submitted to Jordan's advocacy site by parents and children. She was trying to tear down their statements, asking, "Where do they say they actually visualized it or heard the comments?" I replied, "I can't say any more than what they typed in text messages." I added, " If you want the exact meaning, then you're going to have to do a deposition of them; I can't put words in their mouth."

Then the attorney submitted another item for evidence. It was a note from Jordan to his friend Brian, and it was another suicide note, written two weeks prior to him trying to take his life and before the final suicide note he left for everyone to see. I began reading, and tears filled my eyes, but I fought them from falling. If I had only known, I would have been able to take him away from there and gotten him help. They said, "He wrote this two week prior to him actually committing suicide; he tried taking Tylenol but got sick and threw up." They went on, "Brian said he took him seriously but initially thought he was kidding and that he turned the note into the principal's office two weeks after he died." The attorney asked me if I ever knew about the note or that he had given Brian the note. I stated, "No! I did not." I did say that Brian left a message on Jordan's site a while after his death and told me Jordan mentioned something and that he was sorry for not taking him seriously. I told Brian, "It wasn't your fault; you didn't know what to do, and I'm sure Jordan felt like the school would have ignored it like they do everything else." I didn't tell the attorney that part, because she probably would have objected based on the claim this was leading the person or a statement of opinion and not fact.

Then the attorney began asking how close I was with Jordan and whether he was in sports or involved with other events, and I replied, "Yes." I told her Jordan would try out for anything to be a part of something. He was in Cub Scouts, Boy Scouts, Little League baseball for five years, and Little League football for three years. The attorney then asked, "Did you attend any of his games?" I said, "Yes, but I could only make it to about a dozen games in all and one freshman football game." I told her ever since Jordan was a toddler, he had always wanted to live with me, and he was like a little monkey, hanging on me wherever I went. I told the attorney that the year of his death, we went to three concerts (Bon Jovi, Kenny Chesney, Ted Nugent, Poison, and Mötley Crüe), and we went to about eight baseball games in total. I also mentioned the bicycle rides we went on and that he rode seventy-three miles in six hours with me, and he was very proud of his accomplishment, as well as how I taught him how to ride a 250 Enduro road bike.

The attorney then submitted another document as an exhibit. It was an English paper Jordan wrote for his English 2 class. The attorney asked, "Have you ever seen this paper?" I replied, "No!" The attorney allowed my attorney and me to read over it, and the tears filled my eyes even more; I tried holding them back, but some broke though and ran down my face. I don't know how I made it through the reading without breaking down, but I was holding it all back for a later time away from the attorney representing the school district, not wanting them to see me weak and unable to continue on. The story he wrote was about the best summer of his life, one he spent with Dad going to so many places and learning to ride a dirt bike.

Then the school's attorney asked me if Jordan was heterosexual or something else and whether he ever had nude pictures on his electronic devices, and if so, if the pictures were of women or men. I stated to the attorney, "Yes! He has been caught with nude pictures of women on his iPod by his mother; they were of very attractive women, and there was a good number of them." I told the attorney that I did request the iPod back from her because I bought it for him, and she was stating how disgusting he was and that he was a perv to have all those pictures. I removed all the pictures, and from that point on, he never had any nude photos on his iPod again. I told the attorney that I talked to Jordan about that and that it is normal for a teenage boy to look at nude photos of women, but he needed to consider that he was only going to get himself in further trouble with his mother if he got caught doing it again. I also told him having your items taken away for a while was not fun either, so he agreed. The attorney tried to tear apart anything and everything about Jordan's bullying, by saying, "If he's not gay, then why would the kids call him gay or homo or even faggot?" I replied, "Because Jordan wore his heart and emotions on his sleeve, he cared, and he wasn't as tough as the other boys. Jordan was a boy that wanted to be liked and accepted and would do anything just to be part of the group and accepted by others." Jordan did not want to be an outsider, and the reason I know is because I went through the same things in my life, trying to fit in so people would like me. I found myself trying to be different, going out for sports and toughening myself up so I could defend myself and fit in. I know what Jordan felt, in ways, when he was going through the emotional pains of not being accepted, which he hid.

The deposition was finally over. About six weeks went by, and I received a call from my attorney. He stated, "The federal court dropped the case, because there were no prior reports of bullying and the fact that you filed to be head of your son's estate after filing the lawsuit." I knew it—they let it drag on for so long, and, just as I have told parents, you must request documentation from the principal about your complaints of bullying, because all they will say is there was no written documentation, and that's where they get you. Time went by, and I just focused on work and still fought the fight at work with promotions. About three and a half years before retiring, I had backed the administration into a corner; I interviewed for sergeant and lieutenant and scored higher than the others for both, so I took the lieutenant's spot and finished my career as a lieutenant.

Jordan's Voice

CONFIDENTIAL—SUBJECT TO PROTECTIVE ORDER

Lewis 1

Jordan Lewis
English II
August 21, 2013

The Life of an Underdog

It was a warm summer day June 11, 1998. This is the day my life began. My mother is rushed into the Memorial Hospital of Carbondale by my father to the emergency room. My parents names are Brad Lewis, and Tina Lewis. My mother had me at twelve-forty-three in the afternoon. My mother had me with no intension of having another child, so that makes me an only child. My father had two kids before he had me with a different woman. I have one half-brother who's name is Kyle, and one half-sister who's name is Deanna.

My first memory that happened when I was a one-and-a-half will be in my mind till the day I die. This memory involves my sister and to this day she still regrets changing my diaper. She decided that she would be responsible and change my diaper, but little did she know she was in for a surprise. She took me out of my crib and takes me over to the changing table. She has already grabbed a new diaper, baby powder, and wipes. As she is opening my diaper she is making a baby noise that was her mistake, because at that moment when she had her mouth open she got a mouthful of my pee.

My first memories of school are not that pleasant. My kindergarten teacher was Mrs. Parker, I don't remember much about her class. I have no memory of school until the seventh grade. By then I had more than one teacher a day. I remember a lot of what my teachers were like. Most of the teachers in Carmi's Middle School were women there were only two guy teachers. Middle School was not all that great, I got in trouble constantly, and believe me that

Carterville 210

CONFIDENTIAL--SUBJECT TO PROTECTIVE ORDER

Lewis 2

was not fun. I got to know what the principles office looked like were he kept everything. He always made me read these books that he said changed his life. Some of the books that he showed me were very well written, and they helped me to not get into a lot of trouble. Since reading those books I have hardley gotten in any trouble. My freshman year was extremely great, going to a new school was different, being the new kid and all, but for the most part made new friends. Hopefully, my sophomore year will turn out to be even better.

Moving can change a person's perspective, but doesn't change everyone's. I have moved twice in my life. I moved in the middle of second grade to Carmi. I never wanted to move to Carmi I wanted to stay in Marion, but I had no decision in that move. The move from Marion to Carmi changed my life, because it put me farther away from my father. This ended up with me trying to move away from my mom's to go live with my dad several times. I did this so many times that the police said if I do it again that they would send me to a juvenile detention center. Mom mother still didn't get the hint that I wanted to live with my dad. Eventually, after living in Carmi for six years I moved here to Carterville. If I was living with my dad here in Carterville I would have no reason to go anyplace else.

Your family should live close by so that you can see them before they die or go into a retirement home. That is the way my family is. A majority of my family live about ten to fifteen minutes away. I don't get to see them as often as I'd like to, because my mother doesn't like my dad's side of the family. My parents are in very different lines of work. My father works in a correctional facility in East St. Louis, while my mother works at a nursing home in energy.

People have hobbies and have hopes and dreams. I am honest and likable to a lot of people. I have the same hobbies as people in Carterville. My hobbies are golfing and fishing.

Carterville 211

Lewis 3

Golfing is a great hobby for lots of people. Some people find it boring and some find it fun. Just like fishing, but people here in Carterville actually think that fishing is exciting. The kids here in Carterville have different hopes and dreams. I hope to join the military after high school, then plan on going to college.

Teens say that they are just like everybody else. Some say they are different from people in many ways. Well I am both of these kinds of people. Most of my peers have many interests that I have and I have interests that they don't have. The peers that I have don't usually talk about their hopes and dreams. All they talk about is trucks and football. They also talk about air soft wars that they have with each other.

People claim they have many high points in their life, but there is only one high point in your life. My high point in my life happened this summer while at my dad's. I had the time of my life at his house this summer. We went to Cardinals and Cubs games. We went to several concerts like Bon Jovi, Kenny Chesney, and Ted Nugent. I got to drive his 250 Indero. That he got for me. We went on a seventy-two mile bike ride. I got to play a lot of video games and talk to friends that I have where my dad's lives.

My life isn't close to the halfway point just yet, but it is a few years away. I was born on the eleventh of June in the year nineteen-ninety-eight. I was born in The Memorial Hospital of Carbondale. My mother is Tina Lewis, and father Brad Lewis. I have two siblings Kyle half-brother and Deanna half-sister. I am the only child my mother will give birth to. Life is short so live life to the fullest.

BRADLEY L. LEWIS

This is my description of five categories of bullying:

The Hand of Bullying

Each finger represents a category of bullying.

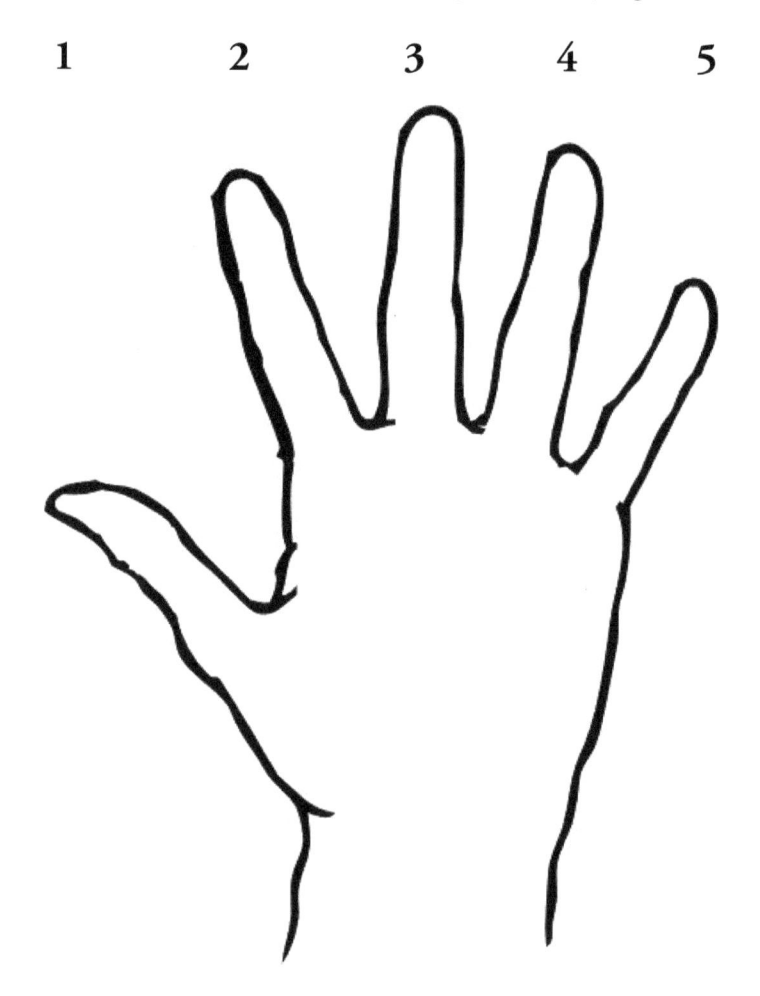

1   2   3   4   5

1. This is a child who is bullied throughout school. He grows up, gets away from the hostile environment, gets stronger, and lives a normal life.

2. This is a child who is bullied in school. Nothing is done, and as he gets older, he is the person who becomes introverted in life, and you see him working in a small cubicle in an office, hidden away; he doesn't have any friends and leaves work and sits at home watching television.

3. This is a child who is bullied in school. Nothing is done, and as he grows up, he becomes the bully in his life, picking on other people.

4. This is a child who is bullied. Nothing is done, and as he gets older and works in society, he is still bullied at work; it gets to a point where he explodes and goes into work and shoots not just the person who is tormenting him but other innocent people as well.

5. This is a child who is bullied, and it is hard for him, and it gets to a point where no one listens, and they ignore him. He goes to school and shoots his bullies and other innocent people. Now, the other course is the child cannot take any more—his life is full of pain, and he leaves a suicide note and kills himself.

★ ★ ★

When I finally heard that everything was over and all the attempts I had made to make changes and to make sure that the lives of Jordan and other children who had committed suicide were not in vain, I got on my bicycle and put my earbuds in and took off, riding about forty miles; during that time, I was away from everyone, and it was me and God out on the road. I began remembering the English paper Jordan wrote ("The Life of an Underdog") and how his last summer was the best summer in his life while listening to "Hey Jude" by the Beatles. The tears started pouring like never before, and I screamed as loud as I could "I love you, Monkey Butt" and continued to sing the rest of the way.

Jordan had a verse on his phone that would come up when he sent text messages and I had it engraved on his headstone:

> And I heard every creature in Heaven and on earth and under the earth and in the sea, and all that is in them saying, "To him who sits on the throne and to the lamb be blessing and honor and glory and might forever!" (Revelations 5:13)

Jordan believed the meaning of that scripture was, "Let all nations sing praises to his name!" *Amen*, Monkey Butt.

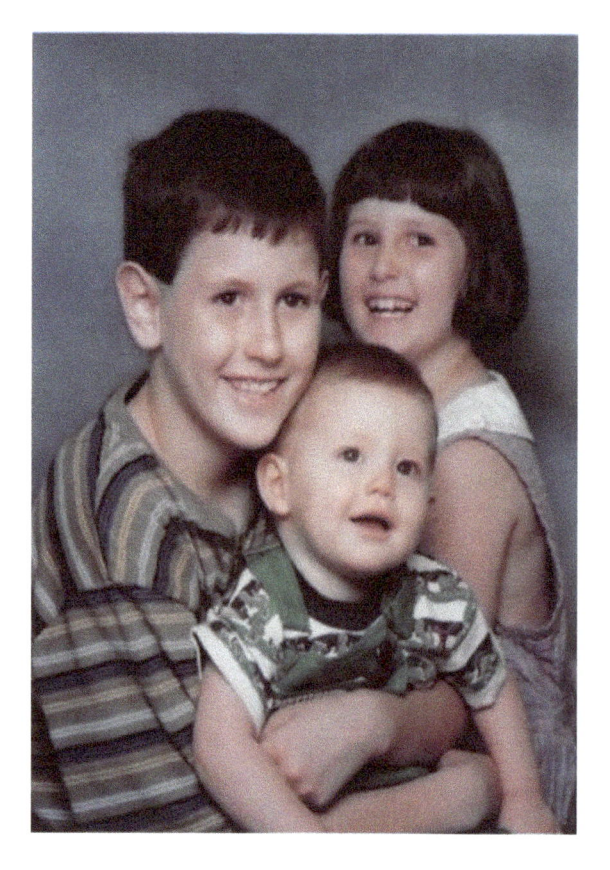

This is Jordan and his siblings.

Jordan's Voice

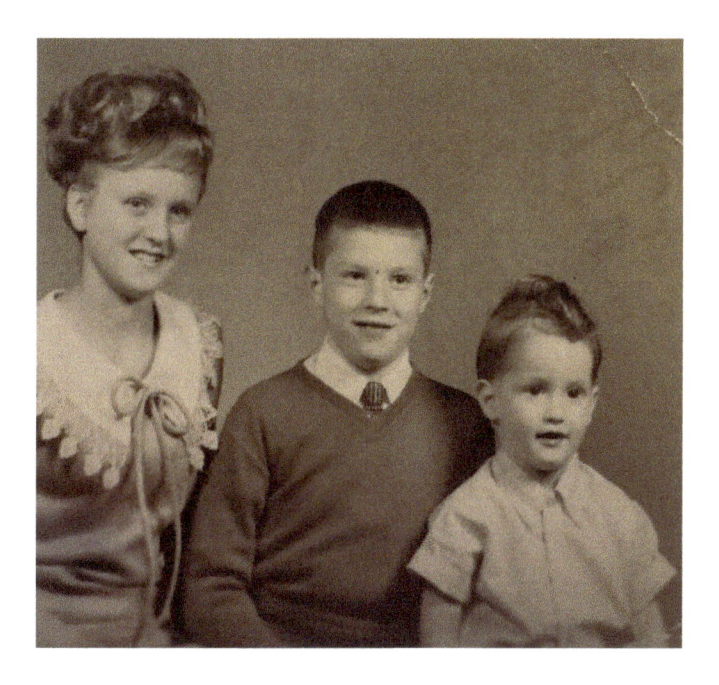

This picture is Brad and siblings.

We begin with: "We the people of this country we call great, in order to form a more perfect union, to establish justice and liberty for ourselves and our prosperity, to ordain and establish the Constitution of America…" These were the words of our forefathers, who developed the blueprints so that this country would not be governed by foreign countries. The Constitution and laws have been created to give the citizens of this country rights but not alter our ways to suit the natural way of life to which they were accustomed. Since the Constitution's drafting, we have seen changes in our beliefs and ways of life. Slavery was abolished, and Black men were given the right to vote, as were women in the early 1900s. Blacks were given equality, as women were given equal rights to men, and then came gay rights and equality with same-sex marriage.

We have overcome numerous obstacles in life in just over 150 years. Why can we not protect our children from physical and mental harm in schools, on the playground, or on the internet? Laws are in place! The definition is clear on the point that it encompasses everyone, leaving no one out. Our problem is, we are afraid to enforce and mandate the laws that are already there. I find that in situations where the schools tell parents they will take care of it when kids are being bullied, after a brief period, it is forgotten about, and when it occurs again and something more severe happens, they have no recollection of any prior events.

We had a governor sign an anti-bullying bill into law in 2014, and his quote in the paper was, "By signing this bill, I'm hoping schools will implement this in their school guidelines and daily curriculum." If you are creating a bill and you are signing it into law, you should not be *hoping* they will abide by it; the law states how it should be. The problem with laws is that there are no mandates, stipulations, or consequences for not following the guidelines of the law. Hence the schools are not held liable unless there are paper trails formed showing nothing was done, but if they do not document it, there are no paper trails.

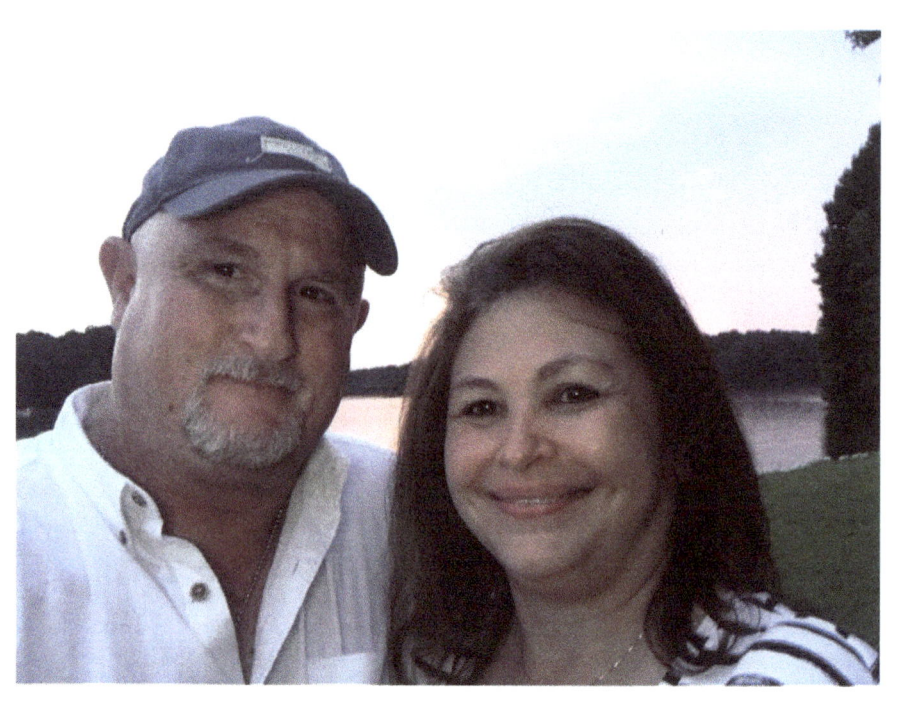

Bradley and Elaine Lewis, 2024

Life of the Underdog

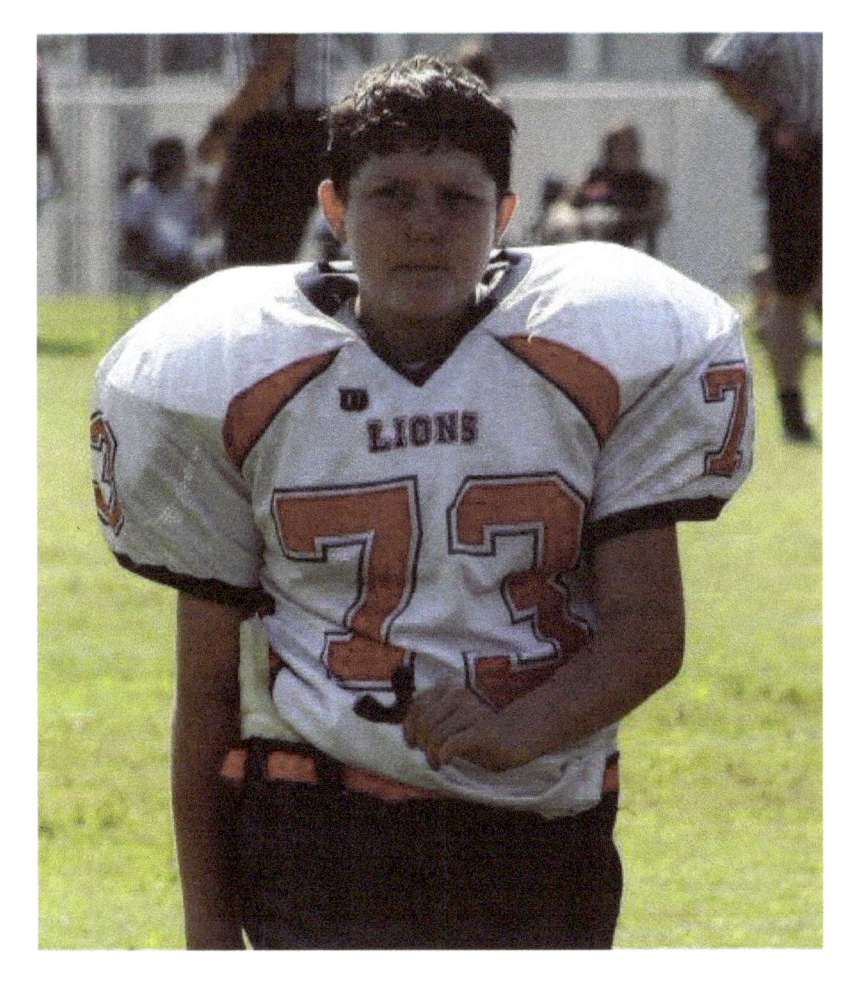

Born June 11, 1998; died October 17, 2011

JORDAN'S VOICE AGAINST BULLYING

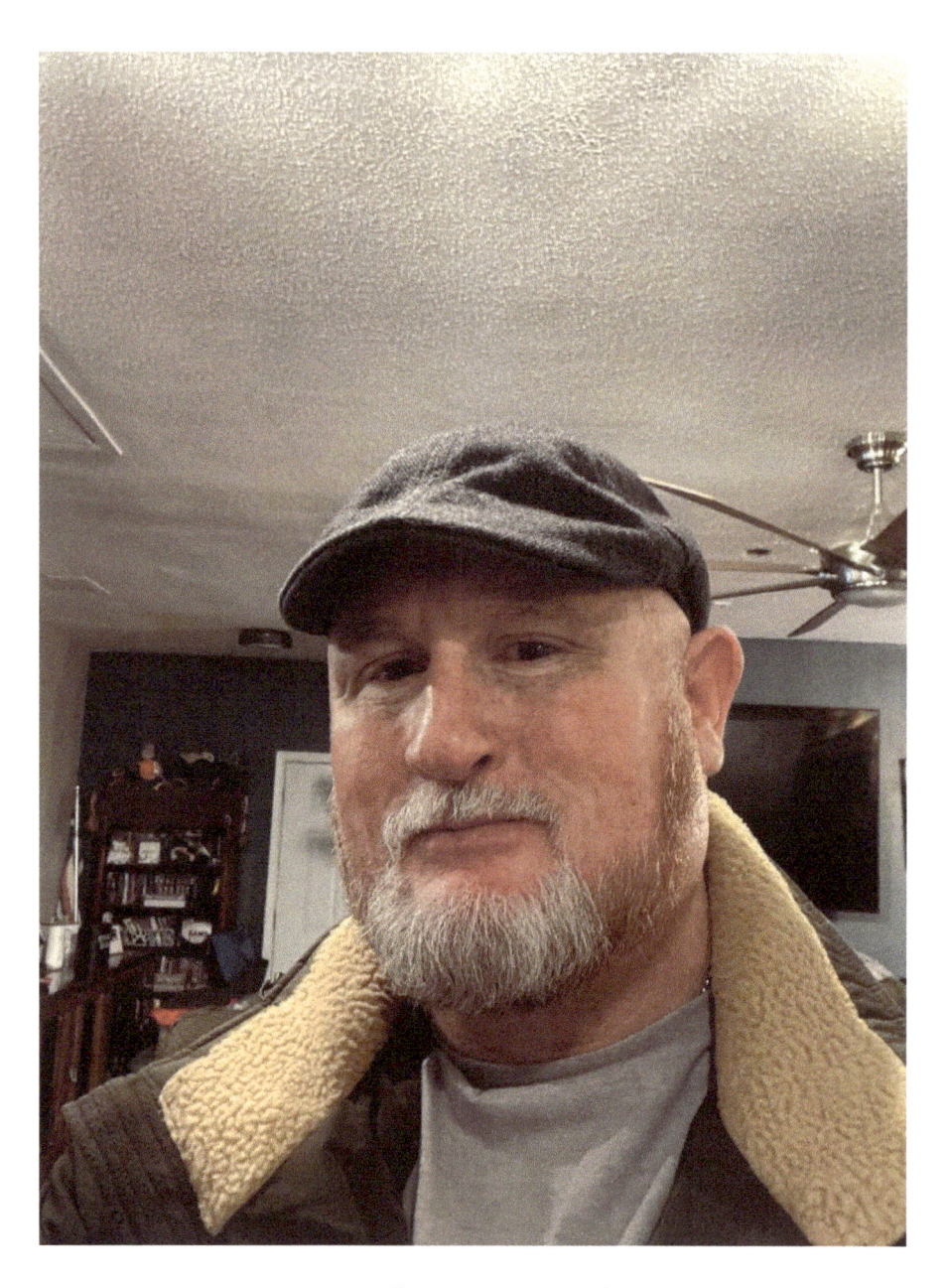

Bradley L. Lewis, 2024